Grahan

4 WEEK
DIABESITY CURE

Cure Diabetes and
loose weight in weeks
with a Keto Diet and
Intermittent Fasting

Disclaimer

All information is believed accurate at the time of going to press but is not so warranted. The publisher shall not be responsible for errors or omissions.

All content within this report is commentary or opinion and is protected under Free Speech laws in all the civilized world. The information herein is provided for educational and entertainment purposes only. It is not intended as a substitute for professional medical advice of any kind.

In no event shall Dr. Graham Simpson be liable for any consequential injury, damages or death arising out of any use of, or reliance on any content or materials contained herein, neither shall Dr. Graham Simpson be liable for any content of any external internet sites referenced and services listed.

Always consult your own licensed medical practitioner if you are in any way concerned about your health. You must satisfy yourself of the validity of the professional qualifications of any health care provider you contact as a result of this book.

Contents

PART 2. THE PROBLEM: GLOBAL DIABESITY

PART 3. FOUR WEEK DIABETES CURE

I dedicate this book to all those suffering from obesity, diabetes, and cardio-metabolic disease.

FOREWORD

Even the title is exhilarating. The fact that diabetes can be cured at all will surprise most doctors; the fact it can be so quick is probably too much for them to take in!

Yet here, in the covers of one slim book, is a fantastic array of tools and knowledge, which will indeed deliver on the title.

My friend Dr. Simpson is a clinician of great skill and experience and he not only tells us the science behind successful remission of one of the world's most complicated killer diseases but he has had years of experience proving his system works. Not only works, it works well!

Today there are over half a billion diabetic sufferers worldwide, almost all of whom are seriously overweight or obese (hence diabesity). *The Journal of the American Medical Association* (JAMA) published in 2017 showed that 53% of Americans were diabetic or prediabetic. Recent research shows that 80% of Americans now have abnormal blood sugar levels. The fact there is such a tide of sickness speaks loudly that the medical profession doesn't really know what it is doing.

The rise in diabesity and the resulting deaths from heart disease, strokes and other related conditions tells us that typical doctors are MIS-managing the problem. A cynical observer like myself might even suggest that it is medical incompetence that is killing the patients, not the diabetes itself.

Because the disease is entirely remediable, as you will read. No-one should die young because of this condition. All it takes is application of real science, not the drug-bound dogma of a profession mired in pursuit of profits over patient care.

As Dr. Simpson tells us, only about 100 years ago, diabetes was a very rare disease (10 out of 35,000 patients). Few people were overweight, never mind obese. Today diabesity is responsible for around 80% of the so-called "diseases of civilization", meaning degenerative and inflammatory processes, such as arthritis, colitis, Alzheimer's, heart disease and stroke. Even cancer was very rare until the twentieth century.

So what changed?

Bad advice, bad science, vested interest and faulty government interference in health matters, that's what. Starting in the 1970s the Food Industry began to meddle with purely medical science, to enlarge its grasp and create more profits. We now have clear evidence that the science peddled by official "researcher" Ancel Keys was deliberately biased, even faked, to support the Big Food giant conglomerates, who wanted to sell us more sugar, more cheap grains, such as corn and more unhealthy vegetable oils.

So we endured the government food pyramid. People were told to eat 60% of their calories in the form of carbohydrates, fats were demonized and even protein was declared potentially "dangerous". The epidemic of obesity we now see was born. Soon a whole new disease—diabesity—had been invented by this meddling and Big Pharma profits from treating this "disease" grew into the $billions annually. All the while patients led unhappy, crippled lives, because they were not being treated successfully, just "managed" until they died. The scenario seems like the plot of a sick and twisted movie—but it's real, not fiction.

The only chance a sufferer has to recover from diabesity and get back to enjoyable health is to get OUT of the medical system and look after his or her own condition, using real knowledge and real science.

That's where this little book comes in. It's packed with understanding of what humans SHOULD be eating and—you know what—it's just what nature herself intended us to eat. If you look at Stone Age societies, including those that were around until the middle of the twentieth century, man was a hunter-gatherer. We were lean and athletic.

Forget the myth that cavemen died young. Apart from being killed by a wild animal, or by infectious diseases just like today, evidence is clear that early Man lived to a full three-score-years-and-ten (70). Not only that but their skeletons were tall, healthy and superb, without any trace of arthritis or other degenerative diseases.

So it's time to turn the clock back. Or rather forward. Because we cannot go on as we are, getting it so horribly wrong that even young children are now developing rampant "diabesity" and at grave risk of dying too young.

Think of it rather as a fake illness, that has been manufactured, and needs to be eradicated from the earth. The way to do that is, of course, to work with the true cause of the problem and DEAL WITH IT.

The answer lies in what we eat on a daily basis. We were not meant to stuff our faces with pizzas, pasta, bread, cookies, candies and cakes, washed down with sodas that contain spoonsful of sugar in every serving.

The result of doing so is that we become addicted to carbs, feel hungry most of the time, over-eat, and guzzle repeatedly, several times a day. It's a treadmill and it is deadly. What do farmers feed their livestock to fatten up the beasts for more profits? Carbs! What does the government tell us to eat? More carbs.

But what will I eat if I give up all those good foods, many will ask? Well the first point to grasp is that you will eat far less, because you won't be addicted to food. Secondly, there are hundreds, if not thousands, of healthy, viable, tasty and enjoyable alternatives.

It's just a matter of cultivating new food habits. And for that, I turn you over to the competent care of Dr. Graham Simpson!

Get thin and live long!

Keith Scott-Mumby MD, MB ChB, HMD, PhD

INTRODUCTION

Diabetes and prediabetes have long been regarded as a chronic progressive condition capable of management but not cure.

I am pleased to report this is not the case. My colleagues and other physicians have been able to reverse diabetes in the majority of type II diabetics within a couple of months and often within one week.

Obesity, also due to insulin resistance, can be reversed rather quickly too but not by following the usual Eat Less – Exercise More advice, but by implementing a High Fat Low Carb (HFLC) Keto Diet and Intermittent Fasting (IF) which is the real cure for "Diabesity."

I will use the abbreviation HFLC (High Fat Low Carb) diet and the WFKD (Well Formulated Keto Diet) interchangeably. This diet is really a lifestyle – a new way of eating that essentially provides a high fat, moderate protein and low carb diet throughout one's life.

Part One gives a short history of diabetes from its initial recognition and its rather infrequent appearance to its common occurrence at first in the more affluent population of England and then America, until it "infected" the common man in every country worldwide. This, together with obesity, is **the** plague of the 21st Century. Diabesity now affects half the global population and is responsible for 80% of all disease of civilization and the majority of health care costs.

Part Two looks at today's global problem of diabesity and dives deep into its real cause and puts to rest not only the "cals in = cals out" dogma, but also several other myths of Diabesity.

Part Three, the greater part of the book, looks to the solution of this global crisis and offers a simple program that anyone, anywhere, can implement with some support from a health coach and video visits from a physician when needed.

In the Afterword, I outline the key elements of the "Four Week Diabetes Cure" and include several studies that show simple lifestyle intervention (without medications) can reverse and prevent diabetes, not only for the individual but also for large population groups. Finally, I have included a few individual testimonials.

Graham Simpson MD

PART ONE

A short history of diabetes

"If we are looking for a dietary cause of some of the ills of civilization, we should look at the most significant changes in man's diet."

– John Yudkin MD

1. OUR ANCESTRAL DIET

As we have recently discovered, the unremitting high prevalence of obesity, diabetes, and cardio-metabolic disease – all conditions that are best described as **carbohydrate intolerance** – are due to our modern Western diet.

To understand where we went off the rails, it is important we look back before the agricultural revolution about 10,000 years ago. As humans migrated out of Africa, we depended on periods of fasting and on hunting and gathering eating mostly meat and fat with very low amounts of carbohydrates. Recent examples of these low carb healthy nomadic cultures include:

1. **The Inuit of the Arctic**
   These people eat 80% of their diet as fat, 15% as protein and a few percent as carbs. Vilhjalmur Stefansson, a Harvard trained anthropologist who lived among the Inuit, agreed to replicate this diet inside Bellevue Hospital in New York where he reproduced the diet of the Inuit for over a year proving that carbohydrates are **NOT** an essential macronutrient for health.

2. **The Bison People of the North American Great Plains**
   These Indians maintained their nomadic existence until the Bison were virtually exterminated. They hunted in the fall after the Bison fattened in the summer. The stored pemmican, a mixture of dried meat and fat, supplemented the diet which again was mostly fat and protein with very little carbohydrate.

3. **The Masai of East Africa**
   Masai would eat approximately 1.2kg of meat, 2 liters of milk and 50ml of blood from their cattle on a daily basis and avoided all carbohydrates.

4. **Indians in the Pacific Northwest of Canada**
   These nomads lived primarily on 3 types of fish: salmon, eel, and oolichan. The latter came every spring in vast numbers; they are 20% of fat by weight. These fish were most prized and when dried became like a candle that could be lit. This mono-unsaturated oolichan grease was much prized by the Indians and fur traders.

**For 2 million years the original human
diet was a high fat-low carb diet.**

---

2. ORIGINS OF DIABETES

- An ancient Egyptian medical text dating back to around 1500 BC was the first to describe this disease as a condition of "passing too much urine." Hindu writings in the 5th to 6th century AD described the urine of these polyuric individuals as "tasting like honey," sticky to the touch, and strongly attracting ants and flies.

- The term 'diabetes' which is Ionian Greek and means "to run through" or a "siphon" was first used by Aretaeus in the second century AD, and he very accurately described this disease:

  "Diabetes is a dreadful affliction, not very frequent among men, being a meltdown of the flesh and limbs into urine. The patient never stops making water and the flow is incessant, like opening an aqueduct. Life is short, unpleasant and painful, thirst unquenchable, drinking excessive and disproportionate to the large quantity of urine, for yet more urine is passed."

- Avicenna (980-1037 AD) mentioned two important complications: gangrene and loss of sexual function (ED).

- Dr. Thomas Willis (1621-1675) made reference to the sweet taste of urine duplicating the observations made 1,000 years before in the Egyptian and Eastern writings. Only in 1776 did the English Physician Matthew Dobson identify "sugar" as the cause of the sweet taste of urine.

- In 1909, Dr. Jean de Meyer suggested that a deficiency of a single hormone he called "insulin" was responsible for diabetes (insula-refers to the islets of Langerhans in the pancreas that produce insulin).

- Fredrick Banting, Charles Best, and John Macleod isolated insulin from the pancreas of cows. Fredrick Sanger, a British biochemist, worked out the molecular structure of insulin and was awarded the Nobel Prize in Chemistry in 1958. This paved the way for the commercial production of insulin.

Diabetes is a very recent disease in humans.

---

3. TYPES OF DIABETES

By 1959 two different types of Diabetes were recognized: -

     i. Type I or insulin dependent diabetes (Juvenile)

     ii. Type II or non-insulin dependent diabetes (Adult)

As many Type II diabetics are also given insulin, this classification was largely abandoned in 2003. Likewise, the age division of Juvenile and Adult onset diabetes has also been abandoned, due to the fact that Type I is often found in Adults, and Type II is now frequently seen in children.

Type I diabetes probably comprises only 5% of diabetics and means that the islet cells of the pancreas produce little or no insulin – these diabetics are usually young and thin.

Type II diabetes comprises 95% of the diabetics. They have excess insulin and usually have increased body fat.

     iii. Type 1.5 diabetes-Latent Autoimmune Diabetes in Adults (LADA)

Due to the body not producing enough insulin (mixture Type I and Type II)

LADA is characterized by: -
- Over age 30
- 1 or more pancreatic auto-antibodies*
- Often lean
- No insulin needed for at least 6 months from initial diagnosis

Pancreatic Auto-Antibodies*

GADA	IAA	1AA
GADA 65	ICA	ZnT8A

Gestational Diabetes is high blood sugar associated with pregnancy.

The majority of diabetics have too much insulin.

---

4. DEFINITION OF DIABETES AND PREDIABETES

Diabetes can be classified according to the HbA1c that measures the average sugar in the blood over 3 months.

Another diagnostic test for diabetes is to measure fasting blood sugars on at least two separate occasions. If the level is above 125mg/dl, this is considered diabetes. A normal fasting blood glucose (FBG) is less than 110mg/dl.

HbA1C	CLASSIFICATION
< 5.7%	Normal
5.7 – 6.4%	Prediabetes
>6.4%	Diabetes

An oral glucose tolerance test (OGTT) is when 75 grams of glucose is ingested and if the amount of glucose 2hrs later in the blood is over 200mg/dl, this indicates diabetes. (The OGTT can be wrong 50% of the time).

A better test is to give a loading dose of 75 grams of glucose and rather measure the 'insulin level' over 3-5 hours. We will cover this test pioneered by Dr. Joseph Kraft a little later. (The 2hr + 3hr sum of insulin should be less than 60 micro units/ml). I wonder if the 20% of so called "healthy fat" individuals would have abnormal insulin patterns with an oral glucose load looking at the insulin levels?

Inflammation and Palmitoleic acid (POA) both predict the onset of type II diabetes. POA is synthesized from palmitic acid and is found in higher concentrations in the liver. A high carb low fat (HCLF) diet will increase levels of POA. POA can be used as a marker for lipogenesis.

Most people with prediabetes develop full-blown type II diabetes within 10 years with the risk of heart disease increased by more than 5 times!

Get your HbA1c level.

5. THE CAUSE OF DIABETES IS TOO MUCH SUGAR AND INSULIN

Although there is a strong genetic component to Type I Diabetes, it is unknown what triggers the autoimmune disease that wipes out the islets producing insulin. This book will focus on the 95% of Type II Diabetics.

Diabetes usually develops over 10-20 years, often with the development of obesity, then prediabetes and finally diabetes.

Hyperglycemia (too much sugar) occurs due to "insulin resistance" rather than the lack of insulin as in Type I diabetes. Once too much sugar floods the body, insulin secretion fails to keep pace with the increasing resistance, leading to hyperglycemia and the diagnosis of Type II Diabetes.

It is important to note that both obesity and insulin resistance are actually protective mechanisms by the body to minimize the damage (cell rot) by the overload of sugar.

Therapy for type I and type II up to this time has been the same, which makes no sense if one looks at the root-cause of diabetes in these two completely different diseases.

Furthermore, giving insulin to type II diabetics makes no sense at all. Insulin and many of the oral hypoglycemic medications both make the disease worse.

This is because it is hyperinsulinemia (too much insulin) and not hyperglycemia (excess sugar) that is the real cause of disease like heart attacks, cancer, and Alzheimer's.

The single best test for "hyperinsulinemia" is that by Joseph Kraft MD (Fact 9).

---

6. THE FUNCTION OF INSULIN

Every cell in the body can use glucose (unlike fructose) for energy. Without insulin, glucose in the blood cannot easily get inside the cell.

All food comes from three macronutrients:

- **Protein** is broken down into amino acids.
- **Fat** is broken down to fatty acids.
- **Carbohydrates** sugar chains are broken down to simple sugars like glucose.

The intestinal blood stream (the portal circulation) delivers amino acids and sugar to the liver (dietary fat is absorbed directly into the lymphatic system as chylomicrons). The liver can only store a limited amount of glycogen after which excess glucose is turned into fat by a process called 'de novo lipogenesis' (DNL). Insulin is the signal to stop burning sugar and fat, and to start storing it instead as triglycerides (TG). When the liver is full of glycogen and fat from DNL, these TG are packaged with protein and expelled into the blood stream as very-low-density lipoproteins (VLDL). Insulin signals lipoprotein lipase (LPL) which signals adipocytes (fat cells) to remove the TG for long term fat storage. In this manner excess CARBS and protein can be stored long term as body fat. **Insulin makes us fat and keeps us fat** (fat cannot be converted back to glucose).

The main stimuli for insulin are sugar and grains – flour, bread, pasta, sweets, pizza, muffins, rice, donuts, potatoes, etc. Insulin resistance can also increase insulin so that ultimately "fat drives more fat."

Insulin is the major metabolic hormone in the body.

---

7. UK SUGAR CONSUMPTION PER CAPITA LBS/YEAR

Obesity and other Cardio-Metabolic Disease had its origins in England. This is due largely to the fact that England was initially the largest consumer of sugar in the world; America followed somewhat later as did other countries.

Increased production eventually made sugar affordable to the common man. Once this happened, obesity and diabetes transitioned from being a disease of the wealthy to being a disease of humankind. The rise in sugar intake per capita increased almost 5x between 1700-1800 in England but remained flat in France. This sugar intake peaked in the UK by early 2000. In some countries like China sugar intake is increasing 5% per year and will produce a tsunami of diabetes in the next decade.

UK SUGAR CONSUMPTION PER CAPITA LBS/YEAR	
1700	4-5 POUNDS
1770	15 POUNDS
1870	25 POUNDS
1970	100 POUNDS
2000	155 POUNDS
2014	150 POUNDS

Through the mid-nineteenth century diabetes remained a rare disease. As the father of modern medicine, Sir William Osler, reported in 1892: of 35,000 outpatients seen at John Hopkins Hospital in Baltimore, only 10 had been diagnosed with diabetes.

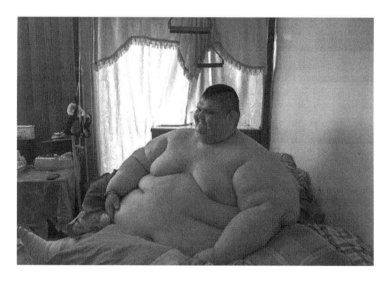

2017 **Juan Pedro Franco**, Mexico, currently weighs 1309lbs and is the heaviest human alive.

8. THE EVIDENCE IS IN FOR SUGAR

We have the data: sugar (especially fructose) is the primary driver that turns on the fat switch causing "insulin and leptin resistance" and cardio- metabolic disease.

> We have causation for sugar → Obesity
>
> We have causation for sugar → Diabetes
>
> We have causation for sugar → Heart Disease
>
> We have causation for sugar → Hypertension
>
> We have causation for sugar → Alzheimer's
>
> We have causation for sugar → Cancer
>
> We have causation for sugar → Fatty Liver Disease
>
> We have causation for sugar → Other Cardio-Metabolic Disease

In our youth we have excellent endothelial (the lining of our blood vessels) function that is resistant to sugar together with low uric acid levels. However, over time in our 30's and 40's due to our continued poor diet with rising sugar and uric acid, the average person puts on 1-2 pounds per year. Thus, we see the emergence of the disease of civilization: obesity- prediabetes- diabetes, and all cardio-metabolic disease.

It's time we do something about this, as more than 50% of all healthcare expenditures are now related to the overconsumption of sugar and grains killing people worldwide.

Peter Cleave and John Yudkin, two of the most famous British researchers in the early 1960's, first suggested that sugar and grains caused not just diabetes and heart disease but the entire cluster of chronic disease we see today.

Avoid sugar completely – it is a toxic substance.

---

9. WHAT EXACTLY IS INSULIN RESISTANCE?

Increased insulin makes us fat and keeps us fat. Increased insulin comes primarily from sugar and grains (and most processed food) that are the cause of high blood sugar levels.

When blood sugar rises, insulin is released from the pancreas repeated over and over again the cells of the body fail to respond to the insulin, and they become "insulin resistant". This leads to further rises in blood sugar and insulin, inflammation of your 50,000 miles of blood vessels throughout your body, and the growth of visceral deep abdominal fat.

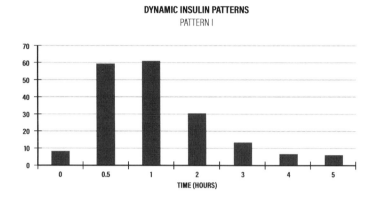

THE ONLY NORMAL INSULIN PATTERN

DYNAMIC INSULIN PATTERNS
PATTERN I

Obesity and most chronic disease seen today throughout the world is due to this "insulin resistance." For example, if you do not correct your diet, the beta cells of your pancreas become exhausted and burn-out which results in diabetes and other metabolic-diseases. A second major problem is when the high sugar reacts with protein in your body, it causes "glycation" and rusts important organs like your blood vessels (heart disease), skin (age spots and wrinkles), eye (cataracts), cartilage (arthritis), kidneys (renal failure), brain (dementia) - all signs of advanced aging reflected in the advanced glycation end-products or AGE theory of aging.

Joseph Kraft, MD and other researchers believe that 100% of people with heart disease have "insulin resistance"; cardiologists acknowledge that 75% have diabetes or pre-diabetes. Kraft showed that the other 25% are not properly diagnosed as you need to load the client with glucose and measure 3-5 hr insulin levels, not the usual (OGTT) wrong in 50% of cases. Sugar and insulin, not cholesterol, cause heart disease (Kraft did more than 15,000 dynamic insulin assays). Hormone levels are usually low. The brief pulse of a hormone is usually over long before resistance has a chance to develop. For resistance to develop, two essential factors are required: high hormonal levels and a constant stimulus with continuous high sugar intake, hyperinsulinemia drives this vicious cycle. Hyperinsulinemia leads to insulin resistance which leads to worsening hyperinsulinemia. **Hyperinsulinemia is the root cause of insulin resistance, obesity, and diabetes – "DIABESITY" are manifestations of the same underlying problem: Hyperinsulinemia.**

**Hyperinsulinemia is determined by direct measurement.
Insulin Resistance is a concept of insulin production.**

---

10. NOT ALL CARBOHYDRATES ARE EQUAL

The **Glycemic Index** (GI) is a relative ranking of carbohydrate in foods according to how they affect blood glucose levels.

Carbohydrates with a low GI value (55 or less) are more slowly digested, absorbed, and metabolized. They cause a lower and slower rise in blood glucose and, therefore insulin levels.

The **Glycemic load** is a ranking system for carbohydrate-rich food that measures the amount of carbohydrates in a serving of food.

Foods with a glycemic load (GL) under 10 are considered lower-GL foods and have little impact on your blood sugar; between 10 and 20 moderate-GL foods with moderate impact on blood sugar, and above 20 high-GL foods that tend to cause high blood sugar spikes.

Carrots are an example of a low GL food. Many people think carrots will raise their blood sugar a lot, but it's not true. That's because although carrots have a high GI of 71, what most people don't know, is that the GL for carrots is only 6. Therefore, unless you're going to eat a pound and a half of carrots in one sitting, an average sitting of carrots will have very little impact on blood glucose levels. That said, juicing carrots – which means consuming more carrots at once – will have a greater impact on blood glucose.

Studies show that starchy carb foods have different effects on blood sugar after eating, depending on the rate of absorption. A low GI and GL diet has been shown to lower blood sugar and insulin. Studies have shown lower rates of heart disease, cancer, and improvement in obesity and diabetes.

Recent research shows that individuals respond differently to a particular food - I might have a high glucose (and insulin) response to a pint of Ben and Gerry's ice cream while you may have a normal sugar and insulin level.

Look for low GI and GL foods.

11. DIET DRINKS AND ARTIFICIAL SWEETENERS

The first diet drink was made in Brooklyn, New York: a sugar free ginger ale called NoCal designed for diabetics. The second was Diet Rite in Atlanta, 1958.

In 1962, Diet Dr Pepper was launched. In 1963, Coca-Cola released Tab and Fresca and Diet Pepsi the following year. Diet 7Up was also released but removed later due to a ban on cyclamate. Coca-Cola released Diet Coke in 1982.

Saccharin was discovered in 1879 from a Coal-tar derivative, Aspartame (nutra sweet) in 1965 (200x sweeter than sucrose.) Over 6000 artificially sweetened products exist and at least 25-30% of the US population routinely ingests these chemicals.

Agave (made from agave plants) is 80% fructose – this and Stevia are no better than sugar. Erythritol and many other sugar alcohols will also bump insulin levels.

You should avoid all the artificial sweeteners due to:
1. you are more likely to gain weight
2. increased risk of heart attacks and stroke
3. increased risk of metabolic syndrome
4. insulin is increased by all artificial sweeteners
5. artificial sweeteners also increase cravings and appetite
6. artificial sweeteners hurt your microbiome

Since microbes in our gut have evolved with us over hundreds of thousands of years, they are unable to deal with artificial sweeteners. In one study from Duke University, a single packet of Splenda upset the ecology of the gut for more than 8 months – it's analogous to throwing a hand grenade into the gut.

Avoid all artificial sweeteners.

---

12. FRUCTOSE IS THE MOST TOXIC SUGAR

High Fructose Corn Syrup (HFCS) was developed in the 1960's as a liquid sugar. Its attraction – it was cheap! Soon it made its way into almost every processed food as well as sodas. Fructose produces a mild insulin response due to its low GI and was thought initially to be safe. How wrong we were? The increase in obesity mirrored the rise of high fructose corn syrup.

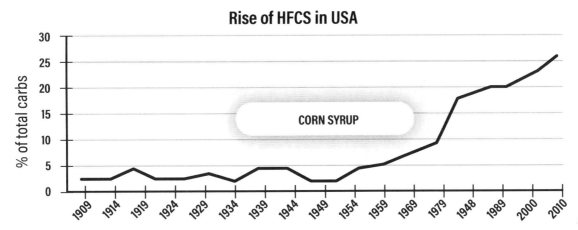

Table sugar (sucrose) is a 50:50 mix of glucose and fructose and carries a one-two punch. Glucose, a refined carb, stimulates insulin while fructose causes fatty liver that produces insulin resistance which also increases insulin levels that causes further insulin resistance.

You **must** remove all added SUGAR from your diet if you are insulin resistant.

Glucose is metabolized differently than **Fructose** in the body.

Glucose - primarily in the circulation regulated by insulin, goes to all cells: ↑ ATP

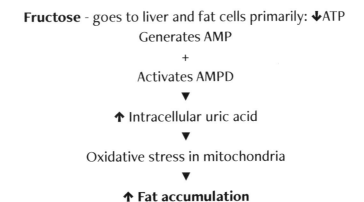

Fructose - goes to liver and fat cells primarily: ↓ATP
Generates AMP
+
Activates AMPD
▼
↑ Intracellular uric acid
▼
Oxidative stress in mitochondria
▼
↑ **Fat accumulation**

Fructose overconsumption leads directly to insulin resistance.

---

13. AVOID ALL FAST FOODS

McDonald's was the first fast-food restaurant to use the assembly line system in the early 1950's. Fast-food is a mass-produced food that is prepared quicker than traditional foods and of lower nutritional value-most often with frozen, preheated or precooked ingredients ready for take-out.

Eating fast-food has been linked to obesity, diabetes, cancer, and depression. Most fast foods are high in trans fats, sugar, salt, and calories.

The global fast-food market is a multibillion dollar business. McDonald's is in 136 countries, Burger King in more than 95 countries, KFC in 128 countries, and Pizza Hut in over 100 countries.

Fast food restaurants have come under criticism for negative health effects, animal cruelty, worker exploitation, cultural degradation via shifts in people's eating patterns away from traditional meals.

10 Worst Effects of Fast-Food Restaurants

1. Obesity (+ NAFLD)
2. Type II Diabetes
3. Heart Disease
4. Cancer
5. Autoimmune Disease (leaky-gut)
6. Increased acne, ulcers et al
7. Main source of Transfats
8. Lacks many Nutrients
9. Waste of Money
10. Lack of Family Gatherings

If you have Diabesity, do not consume fast foods.

---

14. BIG FOOD – AVOID ALL PROCESSED FOOD

There are two types of processed foods:

1. **Mechanical Processing** e.g. minced meat or sliced apples (OK)
2. **Chemical Processing** e.g. Cocoa Puffs or Fritos (Toxic)

Although trans fats were invented in the 1890's, they entered the food supply in the 1910's (for example, Nathans hotdogs and Aunt Jemima's syrup).

Processed food, in addition to trans-fats, are loaded with added sugar or its evil twin fructose that we know is toxic. They are cheaper than real food as corn, wheat, and soy- the main ingredients of these foods- are subsidized by governments.

Before the development of agriculture 10,000 years ago, the dietary choices would have been limited to minimally processed wild plants and animal food.

Dairy products, cereals, refined sugars, refined vegetable oils, and alcohol make up more than 72% of the total energy consumed by most people in the USA and many other developed countries. These foods would have contributed to little or none of the energy in the typical preagricultural human.

Cookies, cakes, baked goods, breakfast cereals, bagels, rolls, muffins, crackers, chips, snack foods, pizza, soft drinks, candy, ice-cream, condiments, and salad dressings dominate most diets today. These foods adversely affect the: (1) glycemic load (GL); (2) fatty-acid consumption; (3) macronutrient composition; (4) micronutrient density; (5) acid-base balance; (6) sodium-potassium ratio; and (7) fiber content. These 7 factors are primary responsible for the Diabesity Pandemic!

Today we eat mostly "fake food" -90% of which is made and sold to us by just 10 Big Food Conglomerates:

1. Kraft
2. Nestle
3. PepsiCo
4. Proctor and Gamble
5. Unilever
6. Coca-Cola
7. Conagra
8. Dole
9. General Mills
10. Hormel

Eat only REAL FOOD.

---

15. BIG PHARMA - AVOID ALL DRUGS AND OTC DRUGS

Already in 2012, more than 50% of Americans had diabetes or prediabetes. In 2010, the definition of type II diabetes was broadened ostensibly for earlier diagnosis and treatment. Nine (9) of the Fourteen (14) outside experts on the panel that made these recommendations were employed by Big-Pharma.

Almost 1/3 of all diabetics in the USA take insulin. I will show insulin is essential for type I diabetics but not type II who have excess insulin!

The Diabetes Control and Complication Trials (DCCT,1983-2005) showed significant benefits in type I diabetes when 'glucotoxicity' (high sugars) were targeted, **BUT** this target of lowering blood sugars in type II did not have the same health benefits as published in the:

- United Kingdom Prospective Diabetes Study (UKPDS)
- Action to Control Cardiac Risk Factors in Diabetes (ACCORD)
- Diabetes and Vascular Disease Controlled Evaluation (ADVANCE)
- Veterans Affairs Diabetes Trial (VADT)

Several other trials also concluded that type II diabetes treated with traditional means including insulin, metformin, sulfonylureas, thiazolidinediones aimed at lowering sugar had no significant benefit in morbidity or mortality – in fact, in some cases treated patients did far worse.

This point reinforces that you treat type II diabetes, a diet and excess insulin problem, with a dietary approach which is the only way to cure diabetes and improve health. I believe that all drugs suggested to you be carefully researched, not just diabetic medications.

The average senior citizen in the US is taking sixteen different medications, most of which they don't need. Remember physicians are the third leading cause of death after heart disease and cancer (Published in the Journal of the American Medical Association) often due to "correctly prescribed" medications.

Avoid all drugs when possible.

---

16. BE AWARE OF THE ROLE OF GOVERNMENT

Before 1920 most agricultural subsidies in the US focused on farm development through programs that homesteaded farms. The subsidies today have evolved from the 1922 Grain Act, the 1929 grain marketing act and later in the 1930's the agricultural adjustment act.

There is a huge discrepancy between what government suggests we eat and what they subsidize, billions of dollars each year. This includes 84$ billion for corn, 35$ billion for wheat and 28$ billion for soy bean which go primarily to livestock or used as artificial sweeteners or other additives in processed foods.

Government in effect subsidizes the diabesity epidemic!

Fruits and vegetables do not have to be more expensive than a corn-laden chicken nugget or corn syrup sweetened soda drink.

As we will see the Governments Dietary Guidelines of 1980 that gave birth to the food pyramid was probably the biggest single debacle that was responsible for the diabesity pandemic.

Diabesity due to unhealthy diets is also the fastest growing non-communicable disease (NCD) in Australia (as in most countries). An article in the Medical Journal of Australia proposed that a paradigm shift from personal responsibility to shared responsibility be made that called on government to take regulatory actions that could modify the preventable dietary risk factors of diabesity at the population level. These regulatory actions should include:

1. Implementing a mandatory front-of-pack food-labelling system.
2. Restricting children exposure to junk food advertising.
3. Strengthening co-regulatory structures for food reformulation.
4. Taxing sugar-sweetened carbonated beverages.

Governments have a duty to protect the population from risks that may lead to disability and premature death. Achieving this on a population wide scale often requires the use of laws and regulations (NCD's account for 85% of Australia's disease burden).

Educate yourself about the Role Government plays in your health.

---

17. AVOID TRANS-FATS

Proctor and Gamble introduced Crisco to consumers in 1911 to provide an economical alternative to animal fat and butter. This vegetable shortening was the first manufactured product to contain trans-fat.

The synthesis of hydrogenated compounds originated in the 1890's when French chemist Paul Sabatier discovered metal catalysts could be used to precipitate a hydrogenation reaction. Partially hydrogenated fat is produced by adding hydrogen (H_2) to vegetable oil thus converting liquid fat to semi-solid fat.

This allowed a stable form of fat to extend shelf life. By 1980 most manufacturers and restaurants stopped using tallow and lard and replaced them with trans-fats.

Trans-fats carry a much higher risk for heart disease not only by increasing oxidized LDL cholesterol and lowering HDL, but trans-fats also increase insulin resistance and type II diabetes.

FOODS CONTAINING TRANS FATS
- Margarine
- Potato chips
- Pizza dough
- Crackers
- Pie Crusts
- Cookies
- Doughnuts
- French fries
- Fried chicken
- Packaged foods with "partially hyd fats"
- Energy bars
- Cakes (and cake mix and frosting)
- Vegetable oils
- Microwave popcorn
- Breakfast sandwiches
- Cream filled candies

Avoid all Trans-fats.

---

18. AVOID PESTICIDES, HERBICIDES AND FUNGICIDES

Pesticides, fungicides, herbicides: All of them contain the suffix "cide," which in Latin means "killer" or "the act of killing." The "cides" in this case indicate the ability to kill entities that negatively affect plants, such as certain insects, fungi and plant diseases. Fungicides and herbicides are forms of pesticide. Pesticides are substances that kill plant pests, with "pests" meaning a broad spectrum of problems, including fungi and even other plants.

Nearly 2 billion pounds of pesticides are used in the USA alone. Worldwide this figure is close to 10 billion pounds and more than 3 billion people engage in the use of pesticides to protect the commercial products they produce. Of the 30 most heavily used pesticides, 12 of the 30 have shown associations with prostate, lung, bladder, pancreas and colon cancer, as well as for leukemia and multiple myeloma. Besides increased cancer, both pesticides and heavy metals have been shown to produce epigenetic changes that also increase the risk for obesity and diabetes.

Monsanto developed the pesticide glyphosate to kill weeds in the early 1970's and brought it to market in 1974 as Roundup. This is associated with birth defects and cancer.

Roundup is also very toxic to our microbiome and produces "leaky gut."

Exposure to Roundup increased the risk of type II diabetes by 60% in a study of 80,000 individuals. Roundup causes low grade inflammation throughout the body leading to gastroenterology disorders, obesity, diabetes, heart disease, depression, cancer and Alzheimer's disease.

Eighty (80) percent of genetically modified crops, especially corn, soy, wheat, and alfalfa are targeted towards the introduction of genes resistant to glyphosate.

Roundup is also linked to the global burden of celiac disease and gluten intolerance.

GMO Crops are banned in over 38 countries worldwide including six ME countries.

Avoid all pesticides – buy Organic – No GMO foods!

---

19. C-PEPTIDE TESTING IN DIABETES

C-peptide is a widely used measure of pancreatic beta cell function. Beta cells secrete pro-insulin (immature alpha and beta chains connected by C-peptide) when C-peptide is removed you get the active form of insulin. Insulin and C-peptide are secreted in equal amounts. The degradation rate of C-peptide in the body is slower than insulin (half-life 20-30mins) compared to half-life of insulin of just 3-5mins which offers a more stable test window of beta cell function.

In healthy individuals the plasma C-peptide in the fasting state is .3-.6nmol/L with a post prandial increase to 1-3nmol/L.

A C-peptide level of less than .2nmol/L is indicative of Type I Diabetes.

Thus C-peptide can distinguish diabetes caused by autoimmune disease (low insulin and C-peptide levels) from lifestyle induced diabetes (with high insulin and C-peptide levels). Thus a low C-peptide indicates that insulin will need to be given.

With a high C-peptide level 95% of diabetics can be reversed with a Keto diet and intermittent fasting.

C-peptide can be measured in the random, fasting (8hrs) or stimulated state. Provocative testing with glucagon is the method of choice.

C-peptide has also been demonstrated to predict microvascular complications of diabetes.

**Test C-peptide level in type II diabetics
not responding to lifestyle therapy.**

---

20. US MACRONUTRIENT CONSUMPTION 1965-2011

Data from the National Health and Nutrition Examination Survey (NHANES) shows that between 1965 and 2000, as the twin epidemics of obesity and type II diabetes unfolded, Americans ate more carbohydrates and less dietary fat, just as the US dietary guidelines had recommended.

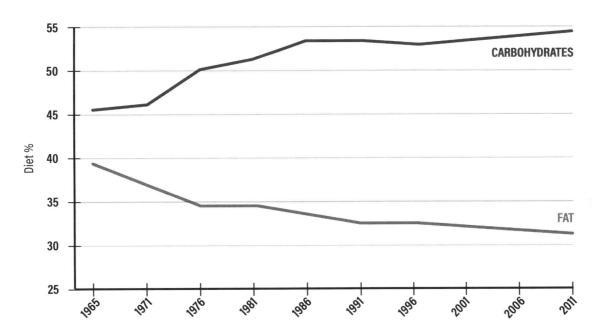

U.S. Macronutrient Consumption 1965-2011

These guidelines together with the changes in the macronutrient composition of our diet, the introduction of sodas, processed snack foods, high fructose corn syrup, the low fat high-carb dogma, Big Pharma, artificial sweeteners, fast-food restaurants, trans-fats, vegetable oils, Big Food, Big Agri and Government **all** laid the foundation for the biggest health crisis the world has ever seen.

**You will relearn how to eat a High
Fat Low Carb (HFLC) diet.**

PART TWO

The problem:
Global diabesity

It is now increasingly recognized that the low-fat campaign has been based on little scientific evidence and may have caused unintended health consequences.

– Dr. Walter Willet
  Harvard School of Public Health

21. THE DIETARY GUIDELINES FOR AMERICANS (1980) ARE WRONG

Diabesity, the Global Pandemic of the 21st Century is the result of two misguided ideas: the Diet-Heart Hypothesis formulated by Ancel Keys in 1977 and the 1980 US Nutritional Guidelines. We were told to avoid foods like meat, eggs, dairy and coconut oil as the theory was that saturated fats raised LDL-cholesterol that lodges in our arteries causing heart disease.

A report released in 1977 called Dietary Goals for the United States led to the 1980 Dietary Guidelines for Americans. These guidelines were to increase carbohydrate consumption to 55-60% of the diet and de-

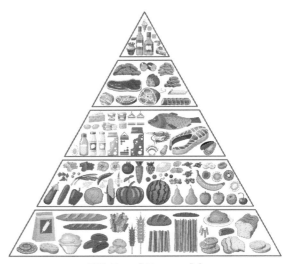

US Food Pyramid

crease fat consumption from approximately 40 percent of calories to 30 percent. The 1980 Guidelines lead to the infamous food pyramid which unbelievably is still being used today.

The American Heart Association, as recently as 2000, preached that low carb diets were a dangerous fad, even though this is how we lived for millions of years. Typical advice was "Eat six or more servings of breads, cereals, pasta and starchy vegetables that are low in fat and cholesterol." To drink... "choose fruit punches and carbonated soft drinks."

This, I believe, is the single biggest reason we find that half the world now has Diabesity!

Turn the pyramid upside down and you have the Keto Diet.

22. THE PANDEMIC OF DIABETES AND OBESITY (DIABESITY)

Many of the factors in Part I coupled with the US 1980 dietary guidelines sealed the fate for many, not only Americans, but people worldwide who followed these faulty guidelines.

Obesity trends in the U.S. after introduction of the "food pyramid"

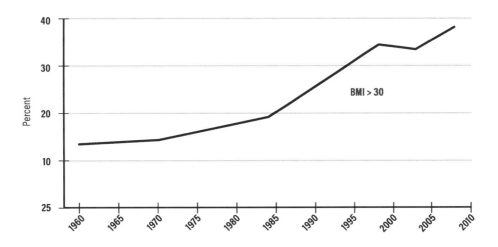

The rising tide of diabetes in the United State

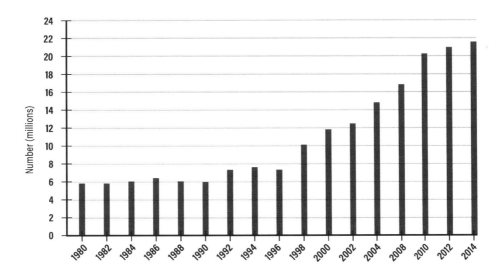

As insulin increases, all people get fat, diabetic and sick.

23. THE 'CHINESE PARADOX' IS NO MORE

In 1980, only 1% of the Chinese had diabetes despite the fact that their diet is based largely on white rice which has a high glycemic index and glycemic load - the Chinese or Asian Paradox. In 2013, it was estimated that 11.6% of Chinese adults had diabetes – a 10x increase in 1 generation.

The Chinese diagnosed had a BMI average of only 23.7% (ideal range). It would be interesting to know rather what the percent of the body fat was in these diabetics.

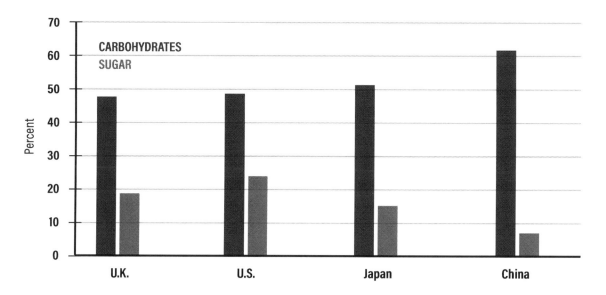

DATA from over 175 nations link sugar intake directly to diabetes independent of obesity (measured however as BMI). The reason for the 'Chinese Paradox' (high carbs but little diabetes) in 1980 is thought to be due to their low sugar intake. However, Asian sugar consumption has been rising by 5% per year (at the same time as sugar consumption has leveled off and fallen in the USA) and promises a tidal wave of diabetes in the next decade in China.

The same relationship was seen in the USA when whole grains were replaced with HFCS. Sugar is more fattening than any other refined carbohydrate and leads directly to diabetes. Fructose in the doses we are currently consuming is toxic - 'the dose makes the poison.'

Grains + Sugar are a lethal combo.

---

24. THE LINK BETWEEN OBESITY AND DIABETES

Following the guidelines from the old food pyramid is guaranteed to make us fat and sick. As you can see from the diagram, fattening CARBS (sugar and grains) increase insulin. This hyperinsulinemia causes insulin resistance, obesity and diabetes (diabesity).

Hyperinsulinemia: The link between obesity and diabetes

FATTENING CARBOHYDRATES ▶ **HYPERINSULINEMIA** ▶ **OBESITY**

▼▲

INSULIN RESISTANCE = TYPE 2 DIABETES

The term "diabesity" implicitly acknowledges that they are one and the same disease. As you will see later from the Virta study, more than 60% of type II diabetics reversed their diabetes, often within 2 months. The average weight loss in the first year was 30 lbs!

With insulin resistance, DNL increases. So much new fat is generated that excess fat now accumulates not just in the liver (there should be none here), but in other ectopic sites, visceral fat, as well as fat in the pancreas, kidneys, heart and muscle.

This ectopic fat is a sign of severe "insulin resistance." By using a well formulated Keto diet (WFKD) – a high fat – moderate protein – low carb diet and intermittent fasting, you can completely reverse this insulin resistance, lose your weight and cure your diabetes. All the key elements you need are outlined in Part III – The Solution.

The Virta study is the first to show reversal of diabetes by simply using Nutritional Ketosis and telemedicine support from health coaches and doctors.

**You must combine a HFLC diet with
Intermittent Fasting (IF) for best results.**

---

25. BODY FAT IS MORE IMPORTANT THAN BODY WEIGHT

I have a particular gripe about this issue. Most of the doctors I visit in different countries do not measure body fat but simply weight (lbs/kgs) or BMI.

I don't believe you can practice Metabolic Medicine without having some idea of a person's body fat percent.

After thousands of body fat measurements, I can say if a male has a body fat of less than 20% and the female is less than 28%, they are often metabolically relatively healthy. This is not always the case, but it is a pretty good screening test.

Make sure you know your body fat percent. You can buy an inexpensive (4 limb measurements are best) impedance device or get it done at a local gym.

A skilled trainer can also use caliper measurements to assess your body fat. The 'visceral fat' is the most dangerous and is a central feature of 'Metabolic Syndrome.'

IDEAL BODY FAT PERCENTAGE AGE CHART

Age (years)	Body fat %	
	Men	Women
20	8.5%	17.7%
25	10.5%	18.4%
30	12.7%	19.3%
35	13.7%	21.5%
40	15.3%	22.2%
45	16.4%	22.9%
50	18.9%	25.2%
55	20.9%	26.3%

The gold standard for body fat percent measurement is **Underwater Weighing**, but it is difficult to locate and inconvenient.

DeXA-Scans – In addition to body fat and lean mass, it also measures bone mass. It is quick, reliable and accurate but more costly than impendence.

Air Plethysmography – or Bod Pod. This is similar to underwater weighing but uses air instead of water.

Waist-Height (Stature) Ratio – This measurement gives an excellent prediction of visceral fat and risk for cardio-metabolic disease.

Know Your Percent Body Fat.

---

26. WHAT IS SKINNY FAT?

Most clients (80%) who are obese have insulin resistance – 20% are healthy fat and often have more subcutaneous fat.

As you can see from the diagram, 30% or 72 million Americans fit this obese category.

However, although 70% of Americans do not look 'obese', 40 % of these non-obese have 'insulin resistance'. They are "skinny fat" or TOFI's – thin on the outside but fat on the inside. In fact, more people (84 million) are insulin resistant in this group compared to the fat group (72 million).

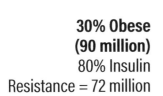
**30% Obese
(90 million)**
80% Insulin
Resistance = 72 million
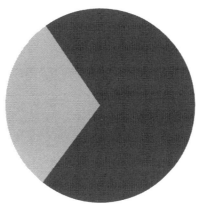
**70% Non-Obese
(210 million)**
40% Insulin Resistance
TOFI = 84 million

This is why you must check your body-fat percent. I am often amazed when a slightly built young girl steps on the body-fat analyzer and I see 38% or more fat.

Mayo Clinic, a number of years ago, published an article that showed many people who are TOFI's also have the diagnosis of Metabolic Syndrome but look very different than the usual obese person with Metabolic Syndrome.

Are you a TOFI with Metabolic Syndrome?

---

27. WHAT IS METABOLIC SYNDROME?

Metabolic Syndrome affects more than one third of the adult population of the USA and was first described by Gerald Reaven from Stanford University in 1988. He noticed a group of risk factors that have a common origin: hypertension, central obesity, high triglycerides, low HDL and diabetes (below diagram).

The common cause is "insulin resistance" due primarily from sugar and grains. Insulin and fructose are the two main activators of DNL.

High triglycerides (increase the risk of heart disease by 61 percent) and low levels of HDL both result from increased VDRL which comes from hyperinsulinemia from too much glucose and fructose.

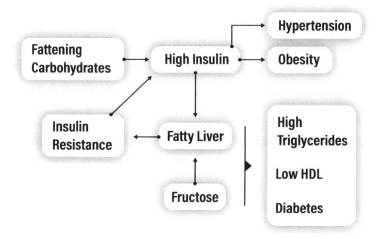

The liver tries to release the fatty congestion by exporting T.G. and blood levels increase- a classic sign of metabolic syndrome (uric acid is also elevated). Ectopic fat accumulates in other organs such as the pancreas, kidneys, heart and muscle. The predominance of fat around the abdomen becomes noticeable as an increase in waist size (wheat belly). This visceral fat is the most important predictor of metabolic syndrome and heart disease.

1	OVERWEIGHT (WAIST SIZE)	MALE >40" (100 cm)	FEMALE >35" (90 cm)
2	HIGH BLOOD SUGAR	>100	>100
3	HIGH BLOOD PRESSURE	>130/85	>130/85
4	HIGH TRIGLYCERIDES	>150	>150
5	LOW HDL CHOLESTEROL	<40	<50

Do you have Metabolic Syndrome?
If you have 3 or more of the above, you have Metabolic Syndrome and have Cardio-Metabolic disease. (Insulin Resistance)

28. CHECK YOUR WAIST TO STATURE RATIO?

The Waist-To-Stature ratio (or waist-to-height ratio) is one of the best anthropomorphic measurements to predict cardio-metabolic risk that shorten life.

Independent of total weight, central obesity is highly correlated with metabolic abnormalities.

Waist-to-stature ratio and years of life lost (YLL)
Adapted from: Jason Fung MD

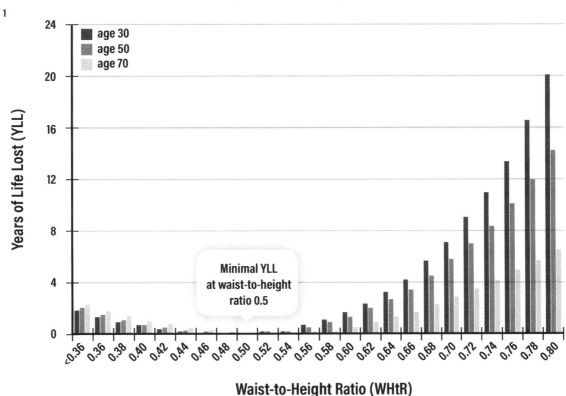

As the waist-stature ratio increases, there is a progression to type II diabetes, heart disease and other cardio-metabolic disease.

Subcutaneous fat, on the other hand, shows little correlation to type II diabetes or heart disease.

Fat within the liver, called intrahepatic fat, is crucial for the development of insulin resistance. Central obesity tracks well with the amount of intrahepatic fat and intra organic fat. Ideally your waist circumference should be half of your height.

Know your Waist-Height (Stature) Ratio.

---

29. NON-ALCOHOLIC FATTY LIVER DISEASE (NAFLD)

Fatty liver can be produced in just 3 weeks by giving overweight volunteers just 2 cokes a day (22 tsp sugar) for 3 weeks. Although their weight only changed 2%, there was a 27% increase in liver fat.

Fatty liver can be just as quickly reversed. A study showed very low cal diets or fasting can reverse 30% of fat accumulation in one week. Normalizing insulin levels reverses insulin resistance.

Obese individuals have 5-15 times the rate of fatty liver. Up to 85% type II diabetics have a fatty liver. The severity of fatty liver correlates to prediabetes, insulin resistance and impairment of beta cell function.

Rising levels of the liver enzyme alanine transaminase (ALT) is an important marker of liver damage often leading to non-alcoholic steatohepatitis (NASH). The amount of fat in the liver does not reflect the amount of organ damage however the fattier the liver, the higher the insulin resistance. You should be vigilant about "sugary snacks"; in fact, all sugar should be eliminated and intermittent fasting implemented to heal the liver.

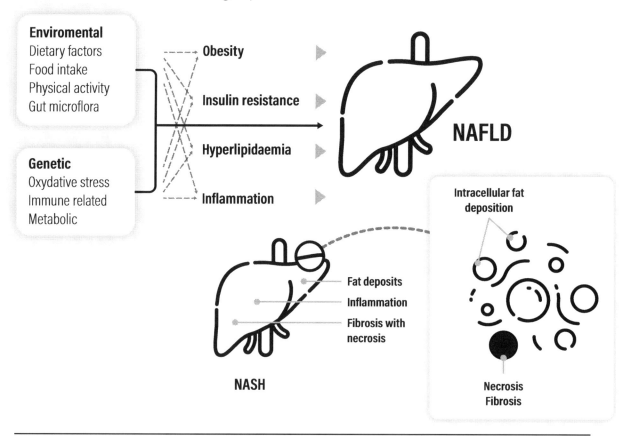

A Keto-Diet and Intermittent Fasting can reduce 30% Liver Fat in One Week.

30. DIABETES AND MITOCHONDRIAL DYSFUNCTION

Mitochondria are the tiny energy factories located in the body's 40 trillion cells. This is where we get our energy from. When mitochondrial dysfunction occurs, our cells are not able to function properly. Fructose is very toxic to the mitochondria.

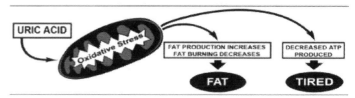

Uric acid Stimulates the Accumulation of Fat

Uric acid affects mitochondria, causing oxidative stress. This results in stimulating fat synthesis, blocking fatty acid oxidation, and reducing ATP production. The net effect is to preferentially shunt the energy from food into fat stores.

FRUCTOSE ELEVATES INTRACELLULAR URIC ACID

The first enzyme in fructose metabolism, fructokinase, consumes ATP while it metabolizes fructose. The process not only generates AMP, but also activates AMPD and intracellular uric acid accumulates damaging the mitochondria. Uric acid is a powerful biological signaling molecule and is recognized as a biomarker of metabolic syndrome.

Hibernating Squirrels and the Fat Switch

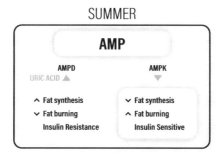
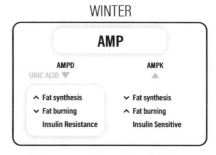

During summer squirrels accumulate fat in preparation for winter. AMPD activity is high.
During winter squirrels switch to burning the fat, and AMPK activity is high.

Chronic Inflammatory Response Syndrome (CIRS), a recently accepted disease (syndrome), produces a low grade inflammatory response often from dysbiosis and leaky-gut that allows different toxins into the blood stream resulting in inflammation and chronic disease.

CARB Syndrome, popularized by Dr. William Wilson, causes a diffuse brain syndrome by also damaging the mitochondria in a similar manner.

Remove all fructose from your diet.

---

31. SURVIVAL OF THE FATTEST

Just as Darwin emphasized the survival of the fittest, there is an equally important concept of "survival of the fattest" (Dr. Richard Johnson). An overriding principal of evolution is to develop ways to survive periods when food is not available. Animals prepare for famine by not only storing fat, but by becoming insulin resistant and pre-diabetic.

Animals activate the "fat switch" that allows them to gain weight and then turn it off. Obese humans have turned on the fat switch and it's stuck in the "on position" that is responsible for Cardio-Metabolic Disease primarily due to the modern diet with its constant supply of sugar and grains.

The metabolic syndrome, according to Johnson, should actually be renamed the "fat storage syndrome". It is not an abnormal process; animals purposefully develop metabolic syndrome to help them survive periods of food shortage.

Anything containing primarily refined grains, potato products, concentrated sugar, especially fructose, turns on the AMPD and Uric Acid (fat switch) and raises insulin excessively. This programs fat cells to hoard calories and a vicious cycle is set in motion with hyperinsulinemia causing more insulin resistance and diabesity.

The "fat switch", as shown previously, resides in our mitochondria; when it is on, we preferentially shunt energy from food to fat (less ketones available). The individual becomes hungry and eats more than he needs , exercises less due to fatigue, and stores more fat! These fattening carbohydrates have initiated 'insulin resistance' increasing metabolic syndrome, diabesity and a host of cardio-metabolic disease.

Understand your Fat Switch.

32. DNA RICH FOODS AND THE FAT SWITCH

Beer, like sugar, is very potent at raising uric acid levels, but this occurs over hours instead of minutes. Beer raises uric acid (unlike wine) due to its yeast content, which being rich in nucleic acids stimulates the production of uric acid. I finally understood why someone watching a rugby game would come into the emergency room with an acute gout attack – most had drunk ½ dozen or more beers at the game.

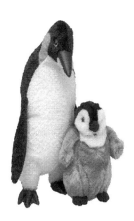

While fructose is an excellent way to increase fat stores, not all animals have access to fructose so that the ingestion of DNA rich foods provide an alternative mechanism. The Antarctic Krill population greatly expands in the spring and are eaten by squid and sea fish which in turn the Emperor Penguin feeds on (RNA rich squid and fish) and doubles his weight in preparation for the winter. He then marches in land where he will incubate the egg laid by his mate until it hatches. During this time the penguin may survive without food for as long as 4 months, burning his fat stores and increasing his ketones as his only food source.

When humans shifted from forests (and the fruits) to a hunter-gatherer society, new foods such as organ meats and bone marrow rich in nucleotides and their breakdown products-purines could now raise uric acid. Thus, foods high in nucleotides and purines can turn on the 'fat switch' in the mitochondria and help both animals and humans store fat.

Sugar, especially 'fructose', is still by far the most powerful trigger to "turn on" your fat switch. Intermittent Fasting will help turn the switch 'off' just like hibernating animals and penguins.

Moderate intake of Umami and Purine Foods.

---

33. FACTORS THAT TURN ON AMPD - THE FAT SWITCH

To reduce obesity and diabetes, you should avoid these triggers:

1. Fructose eg. HFCS
2. Glucose (via polyol pathway) converts to fructose
3. Fructans (wheat, rye etc) gut bacteria converts this to fructose
4. Umami foods
5. High Purine foods
6. Beer, Sodas, Fruit Juice
7. Processed foods
8. Most grains and many fruits
9. Toxins eg. Lead
10. Micronutrient deficiencies eg. Vit C
11. Microbiome Dysfunction
12. Lack of Sleep and Exercise
13. Increased Stress
14. All artificial sweeteners
15. Too many starchy vegetables

*We have taste buds to sense foods that raise uric acid called Umami or the 5th taste.

The Similarities of High Purine and High Umami Foods

	High Purine Foods	High Umami Foods
Meats	High: Organ meats, beef extract. Medium: Lamb, beef, pork, duck, turkey	High: Organ meats, beef extract. Medium: Lamb, beef, pork, duck, turkey
Seafood	High: shellfish, shrimp, crab, lobster, squid, Anchovies, sardines, mackerel, tuna, salmon Medium: most fish	High: shellfish, shrimp, crab, lobster, squid, Anchovies, sardines, mackerel, tuna, salmon Medium: most fish
Vegetable	Medium: Soybeans, peas, brussel sprouts, broccoli, spinach	Medium: Soybeans, peas, tomatoes, red bell peppers, spinach
Mushroom	Medium: portobella, porcini, chanterelles	High: shitake, portobella, porcini, chanterelles
Dairy/ cheese	Medium: Blue cheese, Roquefort	High: Parmesan, Blue cheese, Roquefort
Drink	Beer	Beer

Eating umami foods as a cause of obesity is dwarfed by the much larger role of sugar and grains in the Standard American Diet (SAD).

Decrease all factors that turn on AMPD- the fat switch to cure Diabesity.

---

34. SUGAR AND INSULIN CAUSE HEART DISEASE NOT CHOLESTEROL

1951	Ancel Keys has 'epiphany' in Rome and believes increased fat causes heart disease. (Data completely misinterpreted)
1972	John Yudkin MD from UK shows sugar not cholesterol is cause of heart disease.
1977	Dr. Stout identified the pathology of type II diabetes as vascular directly related to hyperinsulinemia and not hyperglycemia.
1980's	Gerald Reaven MD from Stanford (USA) describes syndrome X – now called Metabolic Syndrome common to obesity, diabetes and heart disease (Sugar and Insulin found to be primary cause Metabolic Syndrome).
1984	Dr. Joseph Kraft believes after doing thousands of glucose/insulin tolerance tests over 25 years that all heart disease related to hyperinsulinemia (diabetes or prediabetes).
2014	Yong (JAMA) reports that excess sugar ingested over two decades shows marked increase in incidence of heart disease (Fructose now linked to more than 78 diseases).
2015	US Dietary Guidelines cholesterol intake poses no health risk and is considered safe and taken off list of 'dangerous' foods.
2016	We have the data sugar (refined carbs) is the primary driver of Cardio-Metabolic Disease and 80% of the health care costs.
2018	We have the proof for the first time (Virta Study) of how Nutritional Ketosis alone can reverse most type II diabetes and reduce the risk of cardio-metabolic disease.

If unsure you have 'insulin resistance', do OGT with sugar load and measure insulin levels over 3 hours. (Fact 9)

---

35. HOW INSULIN LEVELS PROGRESS

Obesity most often precedes the diagnosis of type II diabetes by a decade or more. Fasting insulin can reflect the amount of "insulin resistance" in the body.

Changes in insulin as obesity progresses toward type 2 diabetes.

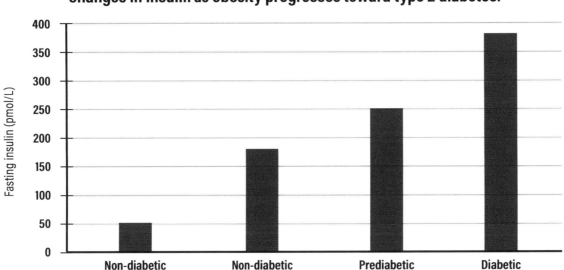

Insulin increases in a progressive manner as shown – from overweight to obesity to prediabetes and ultimately type II diabetes with all its complications.

THE LINK BETWEEN OBESITY AND DIABETES

It is hyperinsulinemia (too high insulin levels) as mentioned that causes both obesity and insulin resistance – for this to develop you need not only high insulin levels but the constant stimulus of sugar.

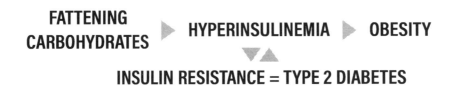

Take a simple fasting insulin and glucose and calculate your HOMA-IR score.

---

36. DIABETES TAKES 10-30 YEARS TO DEVELOP

Cardio-Metabolic Disease that kills 80% of us is primarily due to "insulin resistance." Unlike the plague that kills in days, flu in weeks, AIDS in years, obesity and diabetes kills over decades as the following diagram shows.

This is why it is important to diagnose and cure diabetes as early as possible!

CARDIO-METABOLIC DISEASE

STAGE	TEST
1. Functional Changes 15-20 years	Blood tests Body fat (%) Angioscan SphygmoCor
2. Structural Changes 15-20 years	IMT CAC ABI Angiogram
3. Clinical Event (Western Disease)	Diabetes Heart Attack Stroke Alzheimers

SUGAR AND INSULIN, NOT FAT IS THE PROBLEM

HbA1c 5.5-5.75 (2x CAD)

HbA1c 5.8-6.1 (3.5x CAD)

HbA1c >6.2   (5x CAD)

HbA1c >7   (7x CAD)

CAD = Coronary Artery Disease

Remember: Insulin levels are high (insulin resistance) long before the blood sugar (HbA1c) levels rise as the body is trying to protect itself from the toxic effects of sugar (glucotoxicity).

Take 'structural tests' if you have had diabetes for more than 10 years.

---

37. DIABETES AFFECTS MOST ORGANS IN THE BODY

Several diseases are limited to one particular organ, but diabetes affects every organ.

One of the reasons is the fact that diabetes causes inflammation damaging the endothelium. Obesity-induced chronic inflammation is key to the development of insulin resistance and the Metabolic Syndrome. (The endothelium is the single layer of cells that lines all 50,000 miles of blood vessels.)

As mentioned previously, Diabesity is directly related to hyperinsulinemia and not to hyperglycemia (glucotoxicity). This includes all major arteries, all minor arteries, and all capillaries.

These 50,000 miles of blood vessels thus have a widespread network distributed throughout the body which is why every organ has a potential for disease.

- Diabetes is the leading cause of blindness.
- Diabetes is the leading cause of heart disease.
- Diabetes is the leading cause of cancer.
- Diabetes is the leading cause of stroke.
- Diabetes is the leading cause of hypertension.
- Diabetes is the leading cause of dementia.
- Diabetes is the leading cause of amputation.
- Diabetes is the leading cause of kidney failure.
- Diabetes is the leading cause of nerve damage.
- Diabetes is the leading cause of infertility.
- Diabetes is the leading cause of erectile dysfunction.

The stats are shocking:

- Currently, 2 in 3 adults are overweight (In Hispanics and Mexicans 4 in 5).
- Currently, 1 in 3 are obese.
- Currently, 1 in 2 have diabetes or prediabetes.
- Currently, 1 in 3 adults have metabolic syndrome.

Screen for damage in any organ you are concerned about.

38. CARDIO-METABOLIC DISEASE IS DUE PRIMARILY FROM HYPERINSULINEMIA

Most healthcare costs and human suffering in all countries are due to cardio-metabolic disease from the modern western diet. Chronic disease management until now has not addressed this dietary problem.

CLINICAL MANIFESTATIONS OF INSULIN RESISTANCE

Cognitive decline Type 3 Diabetes	Sleep apnea	PCOS	Malignancies
Erectile dysfunctions	Gout	Fatty liver	GERD
Osteoporosis	Stroke	Cardiovascular disease	Type 2 Diabetes
Atherosclerosis	Hypertension	Dyslipidemia	Sarcopenia

DISEASE OF CIVILIZATION
(Western Disease)

CARDIO

1. Cardiovascular Disease
2. Cerebral Vascular Disease
3. Nephropathy
4. Retinopathy
5. Neuropathy
6. Peripheral Arterial Disease
7. Penile Erectile Dysfunction
8. Hypertension
9. Peyronie's Disease
10. Hemorrhoids
11. Parkinson's
12. Varicose Veins
13. Deep Vein Thrombosis
14. Pulmonary Embolism
15. Migraine

METABOLIC

1. Obesity
2. Diabetes
3. Mitochondrial Disease
4. Dyslipidemia
5. Gestational Diabetes
6. GERD
7. Gallstones
8. Renal Stones
9. Wrinkle's (AGES)
10. Cancer
11. Metabolic Syndrome
12. PCOS
13. Fatty Liver
14. Diverticular Disease
15. Alzheimer's/ Parkinson's

DISEASE

1. Autoimmune Disease
2. Osteoporosis
3. Appendicitis
4. Hormone Dysfunction
5. Constipation
6. Mood Disorders
7. Skin Disorders
8. Sarcopenia
9. Irritable Bowel Syndrome
10. Dental Caries
11. Pernicious Anemia
12. Sleep Apnea
13. Asthma
14. Restless Leg Syndrome
15. Aging

Do you have 'insulin resistance' and the disease of civilization?

---

39. FIVE MYTHS ABOUT OBESITY

Most diets aim to shrink body fat by restricting calories. Here is the truth: virtually everyone who has ever used calorie restriction for weight loss has failed!

They are doomed to fail as they don't address the root cause of the problem:

Obesity is not an energy problem – Obesity is a hormonal problem.

Rather we have activated a "program" – the fat switch – and become fat from processed foods (sugar, grains and trans fats) that cause hyperinsulinemia which causes obesity and diabetes (diabesity).

> *"It is simply no longer possible to believe much of the clinical research that is published, or to rely on the judgment of physicians or authoritative medical guidelines. I take no pleasure in this conclusion, which I reached slowly and reluctantly over my two decades as an editor of the New England Journal of Medicine."*
>
> Marcia Angell MD
> (Long time Editor in Chief NEJM)

> *"Most of the peer review published trial articles are misleading, exaggerated and often flat-out wrong. As much as 90 percent of the published medical information that doctors rely on is deeply flawed."*
>
> Prof John Ioannidis
> (Dept. Medicine Stanford Univ.)

I believe these two quotes from very esteemed physicians give you an idea of the vested interests I mentioned, which includes the medical and scientific community. Professor Tim Noakes was recently acquitted from a lawsuit that took him 3 years and 3 months to defend, well presented in his recent book "The Lore of Nutrition." Dr. Noakes, a friend and colleague, is the foremost researcher on HFLC diets in SA. He was himself wedded to the outmoded HCLF diet until just a decade ago. He was courageous enough to change his thinking when the science proved that sugar, not cholesterol, was the enemy as we now realize.

When you understand these 5 myths, you will understand why most of the advice from the tens of thousands of books on weight loss doesn't work.

---

40. OBESITY MYTH #1

CALORIES IN = CALORIES OUT

FACT: OBESITY IS NOT A DISORDER OF ENERGY BALANCE, IT IS A DISORDER IN THE REGULATION OF THE FAT TISSUE.

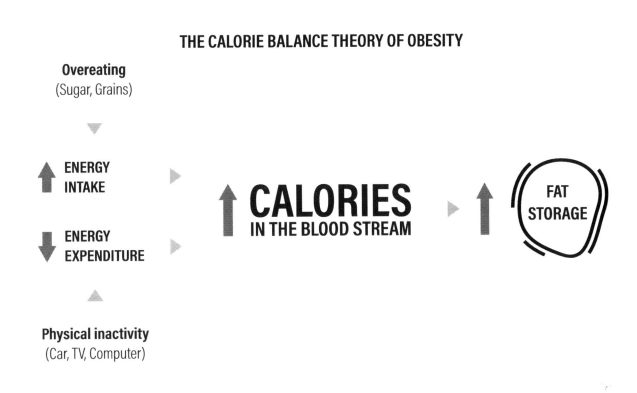

THE CALORIE BALANCE THEORY OF OBESITY

Overeating
(Sugar, Grains)

ENERGY INTAKE ↑

ENERGY EXPENDITURE ↓

↑ **CALORIES** IN THE BLOOD STREAM

↑ **FAT STORAGE**

Physical inactivity
(Car, TV, Computer)

This myth was based on the notion that we get fat by taking more calories and expending less, based on the First Law of Thermodynamics; that it was all due to gluttony and sloth.

It explains why Eat Less and Exercise More does not work – as millions of people now realize.

Forget about calories; fix the diet and hormones.

---

41. OBESITY MYTH #2

WE GET FAT BECAUSE WE ARE NOT ACTIVE AND DO NO EXERCISE

FACT: WE DON'T EXERCISE BECAUSE WE ARE TIRED AND HAVE NO ENERGY

This myth again is based on the First Law of Thermodynamics and is not true. It is "malpractice" to tell a client that the reason he/she is overweight or fat is due to lack of exercise. Exercise has never been shown to help you lose weight. Exercise has countless benefits but weight loss is not one of them.

The "fat switch" causes increased fat storage, which leads to the fat cells sucking up more energy, depleting the body of energy, and causing the individual to be tired and hungry with little or no motivation to exercise.

Some of the benefits of exercise includes:

- Improves gut biome
- Loss of fat (inches)
- Reduce Stress
- Increases GH level
- Increased energy
- Improves insulin resistance
- Lowers blood pressure
- Increases telomere length
- Disease prevention/longevity
- Increases muscle mass
- Improves sex drive
- Increases endurance
- Prevents osteoporosis
- Increases self confidence
- Lowers risk of heart disease

Go Keto, Get Moving.

---

42. OBESITY MYTH #3

A CALORIE IS A CALORIE

FACT: A CALORIE FROM CARBOHYDRATES IS VERY DIFFERENT FROM PROTEIN AND FAT DUE TO THE DIFFERENT HORMONAL RESPONSE IT ENGENDERS.

Processed carbs affect body weight in ways that can't be explained by their calories, but can by "The Fat Switch." Conversely, nuts, olive oil, dark chocolate, some of the most dense calorie foods appear to prevent obesity, diabetes and heart disease.

The Sugar Industries' party line was very different. "Sugar is neither a reducing food nor a fattening food." All foods supply calories and there is no difference between the calories that come from sugar or steak or grape fruit or ice cream." How wrong they were!

THE FAT CELL THEORY OF OBESITY

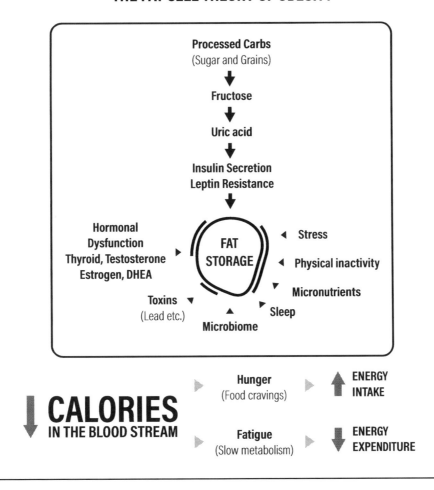

Dietary fat will help you more than any other nutrient.

43. OBESITY MYTH #4

WE GET FAT BECAUSE WE EAT FAT

FACT: WE GET FAT FROM EATING CARBS – PRIMARILY SUGAR AND GRAINS

Another huge misconception was the idea that eating fat caused chronic disease like diabetes and heart disease. This was known as the "Diet-Heart" Hypothesis made popular by Ancel Keys. Just because cholesterol was found in the coronary plaque did not prove causation. Cholesterol was thought as the villain, and we had the whole world eating low fat and high carbs. It doesn't take a rocket-scientist to see what this blunder caused. When his research was properly examined, sugar not cholesterol turned out to be the true villain.

Fortunately, researchers like Richard Johnson, MD and Joseph Kraft, MD, among others, have shown us that sugar and uric acid are primarily causative for metabolic syndrome and Western disease.

Fructose, a sugar in fruits, honey and table sugar, is the master of all food in its ability to make us fat and insulin resistant.

Although there are more than 60,000 grocery items lining the shelves of grocery stores, most of these are processed, high in sugar, grains and trans fats. There are really only a handful of truly healthy products. Shopping on the periphery for meat, fish, poultry, vegetables, select fruits and dairy is where you need to be. The consumption of sugar over the last one hundred years is mind blowing.

Our individual health is determined largely by how we live and the food we eat each day.

You must make friends with fat – Eat Fat – Get Thin.

---

44. OBESITY MYTH #5

WE GET FAT BECAUSE WE OVER EAT

FACT – WE OVER EAT BECAUSE WE ARE FAT

Our major energy currency in our body is ATP produced in our mitochondria. As discussed earlier, the first enzyme in fructose metabolism, fructokinase, consumes ATP (our energy source) while it metabolizes fructose. The process not only generates AMP, but also activates AMPD and intracellular uric acid which accumulates, damaging the mitochondria.

When the 'fat switch' residing in our mitochondria is ON, we preferentially shunt energy from food to fat. The fat cells suck up energy that results in less energy to fuel the body. The individual becomes hungry and eats more than he/she needs, and exercises less due to fatigue, and stores more fat.

THE FAT SWITCH

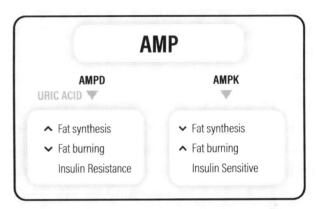

AMP is produced daily during the metabolism of ATP and nucleic acids. If AMP is activated by AMPD, fat accumulation and insulin resistance occurs. If AMP is engaged by AMPK, the opposite results. Whether you are burning or accumulating fat may relate to which of these enzymes is in charge. *Adapted from Richard Johnson MD*

It is well known that people with obesity and diabetes have low AMPK activity. In fact, the number one drug used to treat diabetes is metformin, which works by inhibiting AMPD and stimulating AMPK.

Body fat is critical for health and longevity. Fat is our fuel tank and critical for survival. The body stores carbohydrate in the liver and protein in the muscles, but these are in dilute forms surrounded by water. Stored fat is highly concentrated since it contains little water and has twice the amount of calories than carbs and protein.

Insulin's actions extend well beyond blood sugar control. Soon after a meal, insulin rises, directing the meal's calories – glucose from carbs, amino acids from protein and free fatty acids from fat – into body tissues for utilization or storage. Excess insulin drives fat cells to increase in size and number. What mostly drives this excess insulin is sugar and grains.

An understanding of these 5 Myths are essential to reverse Diabesity.

---

45. THE ROOT-CAUSE OF DIABESITY

The fact that diabesity is global and a relatively new disease argues against a genetic cause. For more than 40 years, researchers, doctors and dieticians have advocated a low fat, calorie reduced diet, and more exercise to reduce obesity with no effective results which has led to our global diabesity crisis. Clearly, we had no idea how to help people lose weight and reverse diabetes. I am pleased to say this is no longer the case, as more and more people recognize that a WFKD can halt and reverse most disease of civilization.

The most important factor in controlling fat accumulation and weight gain is to control the hormonal signals you get from food, not the total number of calories.

As explained earlier, obesity is a hormonal problem, not a caloric one. The hormonal problem with undesired weight gain and fat is due to excessive insulin coming from sugar and grains. This is exactly the same cause for the development of type II diabetes.

No amount of drugs will cure diabesity. It is a food problem and needs a dietary cure.

A high insulin is a signal for the body to stop burning sugar and fat and to start storing it instead.

If our feeding periods predominate over our fasting periods, then this insulin excess leads to fat accumulation → prediabetes → diabetes and other cardio-metabolic disease.

It is worth remembering that Ethan Allen Sims MD, Professor of Medicine (Vermont University) coined the term "diabesity" in 1972. By overfeeding young men with a high carb low fat (HCLF) typical standard American diet, with no family history of diabetes, within a few months the initial signs of diabesity were induced in these young men.

Forget counting calories forever.

PART THREE

Four week
diabetes cure

Every single day, I see patients whose type II diabetes is reversing, patients who are losing weight and getting healthier. This is the reason I became a doctor! I want to help people regain their health, and I want to give people hope that they can indeed defeat obesity and type II diabetes, completely naturally. That's perfect, because patients also do not want to be sick or take medications. It's a win-win situation.

– Jason Fung MD
  The Diabetes Code

46. OUR MODERN WESTERN DIET OR STANDARD AMERICAN DIET (SAD)

As ancient cultures began to implement agriculture, nomadic folk lost much of their wisdom. (I refer the interested reader to Jimmy Nelson's excellent book "Before They Pass Away").

Realizing our current crisis begs the question: Who rules our thinking and beliefs about accurate dietary principles? Is it the academic nutrition community, scientists, doctors, dieticians, Big Food, Big Pharma, Big Sugar, government? If we peek under the covers at where the money and power lie, it becomes clear that these groups discount the science of low carb diets.

The good news is that this is about to change! Although the **Paleo-Diet** gained momentum more than a decade ago, especially with the good research by Loren Cordain and others, it is clear that its 30% carb recommendations did not go far enough to reverse "insulin resistance" now affecting nearly half the world's population.

I believe the **Keto-Diet** will become the major therapeutic intervention in the decade to come that can help reverse our modern day cardio-metabolic pandemic. It is the "tipping point" that will move us from reactive medicine towards proactive health.

As mentioned in Part I and Part II, many of these "power players" helped to get us in the mess we find ourselves today. The biggest scam in the history of medicine is the Diet – Heart hypothesis advanced by Ancel Keys and the absurd 1980 US Dietary Guidelines that encouraged Americans (and the world) to raise their carbohydrate consumption to 55-60% and decrease fat consumption from 40% to 30% of calories.

Try a WFKD for 30 days for proof.

---

47. WHAT DOES A LOW CARB DIET REALLY MEAN?

The Diagram below shows the **Standard American Diet (SAD)** with its 55-60% CARB intake and the **Mediterranean Diet** with its moderate carb diet (35-40%).

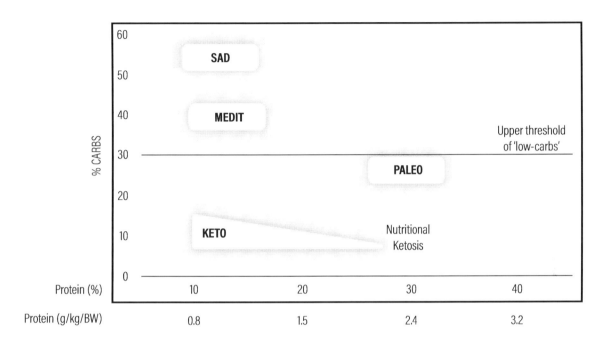

*Protein can vary depending on the individual from 65-120gm

Adapted from Dr. Phinney and Professor Volek

From the diagram, the upper limit of a low carb diet is 30% carbohydrates. The **Paleo Diet** is a moderate carb, moderate protein, and moderate fat diet.

A well formulated **Keto Diet** is High Fat (70%), Moderate Protein (20%) and Low Carb (10%). This is the HFLC diet that produces nutritional ketosis to reverse "insulin resistance", diabetes, obesity and the disease of civilization.

Move toward a well formulated Keto Diet Lifestyle

---

48. THE ONLY WAY TO CURE DIABESITY

The two best ways to predict who will develop diabetes (insulin resistance) in a cohort of healthy subjects are biomarkers of inflammation (CRPhs, IL6, etc.) and the biomarker of lipogenesis (POA) due to sugar overload.

These two processes are linked together by increased ROS production damaging mitochondria and membranes leading to insulin resistance.

We know that insulin and oral hypoglycemics do not cure diabetes. They may lower glucose levels (glucotoxicity) but do not improve hyperinsulinemia, mortality, or morbidity.

The cure for diabesity must therefore be two-fold:

1. Decrease sugar intake (HFLC Diet)

2. Burn off the excess sugar causing lipogenesis (IF)

      BECAUSE

HCLF Eating ↑ insulin and causes sugar and fat to be stored. (↑ AMPD)

Intermittent Fasting ↓ insulin and causes sugar and fat to be burned. (↑ AMPK)

A combo of HFLC diet and I.F. is best to reverse diabesity.

---

49. CHANGE YOUR BELIEFS – CHANGE YOUR BEHAVIOR

In our experience the single best way to change a diabetics belief system is to place a sugar sensor on the arm for 14 days.

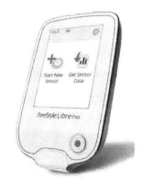

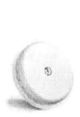

We encourage you to 'eat' and take your 'meds' as usual for 4 days. (Recording 1).

On day 5 you implement the Keto-Diet. Recordings will be done on day 10 (Recording 2) and day 15 (Recording 3).

Sugar readings occur every 15 mins (96x / day) for 2 weeks. Most clients are amazed to see sugar levels drop to normal within 48hrs of implementing the Ketogenic Diet and Intermittent Fasting – this is the key to helping change behavior.

Note: It is important that during these first few weeks close attention be paid to blood sugar readings as most individuals need to decrease the amount of medications when a Keto Diet and Intermittent Fasting is implemented. Physician oversight is always recommended.

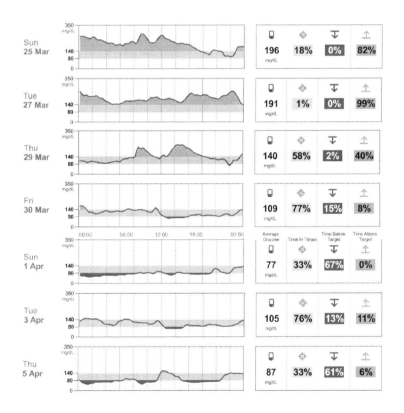

Day	Average Glucose	Time In Target	Time Below Target	Time Above Target
Sun 25 Mar	196 mg/dL	18%	0%	82%
Tue 27 Mar	191 mg/dL	1%	0%	99%
Thu 29 Mar	140 mg/dL	58%	2%	40%
Fri 30 Mar	109 mg/dL	77%	15%	8%
Sun 1 Apr	77 mg/dL	33%	67%	0%
Tue 3 Apr	105 mg/dL	76%	13%	11%
Thu 5 Apr	87 mg/dL	33%	61%	6%

Continuous sugar monitoring can change everything.

---

50. HOW MUCH SUGAR IS TOO MUCH?

The evidence is in implicating all carbohydrates, not just sugar and high fructose corn syrup (HFCS) but also grains and starchy vegetables. Sugar refers to a group of carbs made of atoms of carbon and hydrogen most ending in -ose, e.g. glucose, sucrose, fructose. Table Sugar 'sucrose' is 50% glucose and 50% fructose. HFCS consists of 55% fructose and 45% glucose.

Sucrose and HFCS are often referred to as 'added sugar' compared to the natural sugar found in vegetables and fruits.

The more we use these carbs, the less dopamine we produce and the more we need- similar to the addiction of alcohol, cocaine and heroin.

HOW MUCH IS TOO MUCH?

The literature appears to show that some sugar is OK. George Campbell, MD showed as the intake exceeds 50 pounds per year, we see the emergence of Cardio-Metabolic disease often with a lag time of 18-20 years.

Anything containing primarily grains and concentrated sugar, especially fructose (e.g. processed foods, sodas), raises insulin excessively and programs fat cells to hoard calories by turning on the "fat switch".

Robert Lustig, MD recommends limiting daily sugar intake from all sources, including natural ones like fruit to **NO MORE THAN 25GM/DAY!** (Lustig is a Pediatric Endocrinologist from San Francisco who hosts a great website sugarscience.org).

4gm sugar= 1tsp sugar: **NO MORE THAN 6tsp/day** for women and **9 tsp/day** for men

Average Americans consume 22tsp sugar/day (88gm)

Remember, you only can metabolize 6-9tsp sugar/day; the rest gets converted to fat in the liver causing "insulin resistance" and cardio-metabolic disease.

 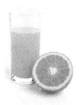

11 tsp sugar   **7 tsp sugar**

Keep your total sugar intake to less than 25gm/day.

---

51. THE KETO DIET – CARB INTAKE – LOW

Low carb diets have been proven far more effective at reducing body weight, waist size, insulin resistance, inflammation, and cardiac risk factors.

Refined carbohydrates, added sugar and flour, increase blood glucose higher and faster than unrefined carbohydrates like potatoes and fruit and cause a greater risk of diabetes.

A well formulated Keto-Diet (WFKD) must restrict these refined carbohydrates to 5-10% of total calories consumed (20 - 50gms). Unrefined foods score especially low on the glycemic load. This distinction shows how many traditional cultures, e.g. Okinawans (Japan) and Kitavans (New Guinea) can eat high carbohydrate-based diets without evidence of disease. Refining and processing plays the key role in enhancing insulin. Fructose plays an important role in the development of fatty liver, insulin resistance, and hyperinsulinemia. Traditional societies eat little or no added sugar.

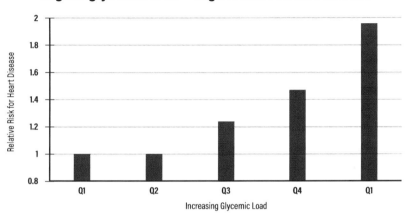

Higher glycemic load = higher risk of heart disease

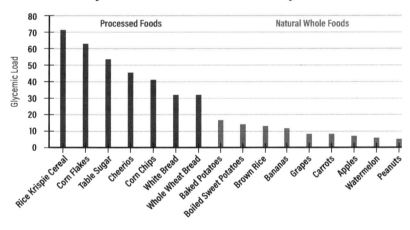

Glycemic load of various carbohydrates

Adapted from Jason Fung MD

Get rid of CARBS – get rid of DIABETES

---

52. THE KETO DIET - PROTEIN INTAKE - MODERATE

We know that fat produces no increase in insulin and have shown that carbohydrates, especially refined carbohydrates, are the worst offenders in increasing insulin, but what about the amount of protein we should eat?

One must avoid eating too much protein as excess protein has a moderate insulin stimulating effect that reduces ketone production. We recommend a daily protein intake between 1 and 2.5gm per day per kg BW, which translates to 15-25% of our daily energy intake. Plant protein has less insulin stimulating effects. Certain longevity experts like Steven Gundry, MD and Valter Longo, PhD recommend more plant protein and lower amounts of 0.8 gm/kg/BW/day.

Protein needs will vary for each individual and needs may increase depending on age, inflammation, certain medications, disease, etc.

Too much protein will also cause lethargy and malaise. The Inuit knew to keep their protein intake moderate. Stefansson, during his yearlong Bellevue experiment, was encouraged by the study investigators to consume a high protein diet during the first weeks of the study which caused him to be weak and sick to his stomach.

Thus, when we refer to the Keto Diet as a high fat-low carb (HFLC) diet, remember that it is a high fat-**moderate protein**-low carb diet.

When protein is digested, it is broken into amino acids. Adequate protein is required for good health and several amino acids are essential and must be supplied in the diet. Excess amino acids cannot be stored in the body, and so the liver converts them to sugar and will raise insulin and decrease ketones. You should avoid processed, concentrated protein sources like protein shakes, protein bars, and protein powder.

**Keep your protein intake to no more
than 15-20% total calories daily.**

53. THE KETO DIET – FAT INTAKE – HIGH

When fat is used for fuel, your body prefers that the majority of it comes from mono-unsaturated and saturated fat. You can eat fat to satiety!

Part of the body's adaption to a low carb diet involves fundamental changes in how it metabolizes fat. Not only does total fat oxidation increase, but the body's rate of saturated fat oxidation accelerates more than other types of fatty acids, driving down levels of saturated fat in the blood. The body stops making fat out of carbohydrates (DNL), much of which ends up as saturated fat in the blood. Understanding this helps understand how a high fat diet, even containing lots of saturated fat, can be very healthy. Even more important is how our body handles polyunsaturated fat when we cut back on carbohydrates. Polyunsaturated fats are components of phospholipids which construct all the membranes that enclose our cells and regulate cellular function. Getting these polyunsaturated fats into membranes is critical for life defining processes like glucose transport (insulin sensitivity), controlling inflammation, salt excretion, blood pressure control, and fertility.

There are three things we do with saturated fats from our diet: burn them, store them or make them something else, e.g. mono-unsaturated fat. When we eat carbs, insulin goes up, which turns off fat oxidation and stimulates fat storage. And when we stop eating carbs or fast, insulin levels fall, fats come out of storage and become the body's primary fuel. Saturated fats do not cause heart disease.

You can carry a vial of olive oil and take 3-5 tablespoons a day or a shot or two of MCT oil a day to keep you in Ketosis and help you skip a meal or two during the day.

We recommend at least 70% of your daily percent of calories come from 'healthy fat.'

---

54. WHAT ARE HEALTHY FATS?

As can be seen from the picture, 70-80% of your cals should come from meat, poultry, fish, eggs, cheese, butter, ghee, coconut oil, olive oil, mayonnaise, and cream which are all healthy. When Bob Atkins, MD reintroduced HFLC diets in the late 1990's, most doctors were aghast believing that this would cause heart disease. Those predictions that this diet would raise cholesterol and clog arteries were wrong. The opposite is true.

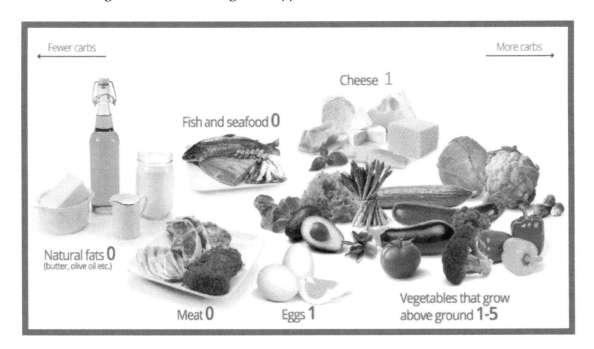

The best fats for cooking are butter, ghee, lard, and coconut oil. Avoid low fat or skim milk, as well as low fat yogurt – low fat usually means high sugar.

Not only did his clients lose weight, but their entire metabolic profiles improved. Cholesterol and triglycerides levels fell, as did sugar and insulin levels, and most inflammatory makers were reduced. The entire foundation of modern nutritional advice was completely shattered.

Many scientific articles verifying this HFLC diet have been published over the last decade confirming Bob Atkins' advice.

Eating fat does not make you fat.

---

55. SUMMARY OF THE KETO DIET

A well formulated Keto Diet (WFKD) will have the macronutrient composition shown in the figure below. It is not calorie restricted. It provides all the minerals, enzymes and fiber that the body needs. Because it satisfies hunger, it is easy to sustain. It is safe and can be continued for decades as it continues to reverse the disease of civilization.

Usually it takes the body at least 3 weeks to become Keto (fat) adapted. The objective is to keep the Ketone level between .5-3 mMoles as shown on the next page. This provides the optimal fuel for the brain, muscles, and body. It will reverse diabesity and most other cardio-metabolic disease.

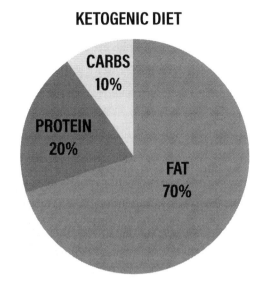

KETOGENIC DIET

To maintain the Keto diet, protein and carb percent stay relatively constant while the percent of fat varies. The fat is what helps sustain us over the long term and is critical to help satiety.

**Contrary to popular belief a Keto diet
can be maintained for decades.**

---

56. OPTIMUM BLOOD KETONE LEVELS

Ketones are potent signals that protect us from free radicals that cause oxidative stress and inflammation throughout our body.

This healthy Ketone level has nothing to do with the life-threatening Ketoacidosis sometimes seen in type I diabetes due to uncontrolled high sugar levels.

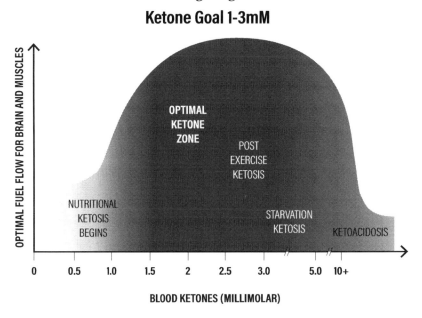

State	Ketones (mmol/L)	
Moderate -carbohydrate diet (fed state)	<0.1	
Moderate-carbohydrate diet (fasted state)	0.1 to 0.3	10x
Fasting (weeks)	5 to 7	
Very low-carbohydrate diet (<50g/day)	0.5 to 3.0	
Very low-carbohydrate diet (post-exercise)	1.0 to 5.0	10x
Keto-acidosis (insulin insufficiency)	10 to 20+	

Adapted from Dr. Phinney and Prof Volek

You must try to keep your Ketone Level greater than .5mM.

---

57. AVOID SNACKS MOST OF THE TIME

Before the 1960's, most people ate just three meals a day. By 2000, most people were eating five-six times a day-three meals and two to three snacks in between. In the development of Diabesity, this increase in meal frequency is just as important as the change in the composition of the diet.

Insulin release with an eating pattern of three meals, no snacks.

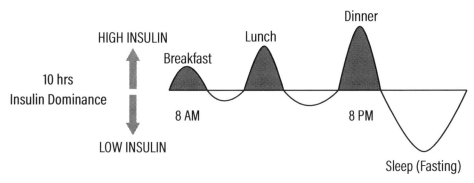

Eating frequently does not increase your metabolic rate or control hunger or keep your blood sugar becoming too low.

Insulin release with an eating pattern of multiple meals and snacks.

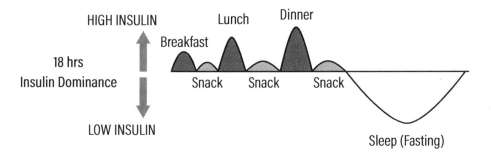

The balance of time spent each day in the insulin-dominant versus the insulin-deficient state has changed greatly since the 1960's.

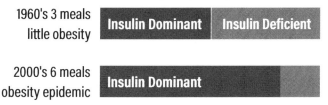

Figures Adapted From Jason Fung MD

Big Food created a whole new category of food called "snacks" in the 1960's, primarily made of processed foods – avoid these!

---

58. A KETO DIET SHOULD BE COMBINED WITH INTERMITTENT FASTING

Fasting has a long tradition in cultures around the world for its benefits to health. There are several popular types of fasting: The weekly 5:2 diet (Dr. Michael Mosley), The Monthly 5/25 diet (Valter Longo) and the most popular, The Daily 16/8 hours diet. The most important feature is the intermittent nature.

We prefer the 18/6 hour IF diet that essentially means having dinner early and breakfast late. When implementing a HFLC diet and avoiding snacks, it is quite easy to get your ketone levels above 1mm. Essentially, you eat in an 8 hour window and fast for 16-18hrs.

Intermittent Fasting combined with the Ketogenic diet is the key to lower the insulin and burn fat. Within a couple of days as you extend your insulin deficit, your body switches from burning sugar (short term) to burning your body fat (long term) and you begin to resolve "insulin resistance."

You can have a 'bullet coffee' or chai tea which has a good amount of fat when you wake up in the morning which will not interfere with nutritional ketosis. Breakfast should always be optional.

It is critical when you are on the HFLC diet that you minimize carbs to less than 10% and keep your protein to 20%. Fat is your key energy source and is the single best nutrient to satisfy your hunger and produce the long term benefits you are looking for. There is no limit to the amount of fat you eat as it does not bump your insulin levels.

It does not hurt to 'skip' a few meals especially when you are not hungry.

59. INTERMITTENT FASTING WORKS BETTER THAN CHRONIC CALORIE RESTRICTION

Portion control does **NOT** work – the failure rate is 99.5%. This does not work for the simple reason that restricting calories causes an increase in hunger and a decrease in the body's metabolic rate.

Intermittent Fasting, on the other hand, produces hormonal changes that chronic calorie restriction doesn't – namely it reduces insulin and insulin resistance.

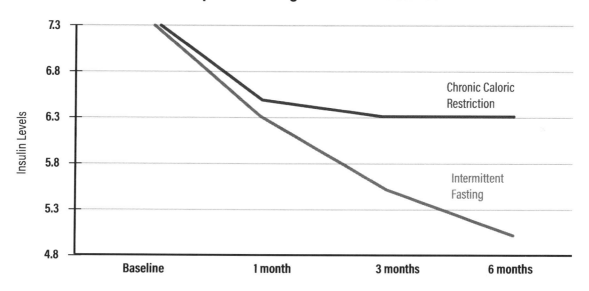

The impact of fasting on insulin resistance

I.F. prevents the development of insulin resistance by creating extended periods of low insulin that maintains the body's sensitivity to insulin. It is the intermittency of the diet that makes it effective.

Remember:
not only is it important WHAT YOU EAT,
but it is just as important WHEN YOU EAT

---

60. WHAT IS KETO-FLU?

It is not uncommon to experience some headaches, dizziness, low energy, and constipation. This is often termed 'keto-flu'; however, these side effects are due to lack of salt and water on a HFLC because excess sodium is lost in the kidney. The remedy is simply to increase salt (at least 2 ½ teaspoons extra salt) and eat bone broth, pickles, biltong or add bullion. Salt is not as toxic as usually presented (See the Salt Fix by James DiNicolantonio).

In the PURE study, over 200,000 individuals in 18 countries were examined. Those taking 5gm/day had the lowest mortality over the 4 year study.

Remember to increase your water intake on a keto-diet and also other minerals like potassium and magnesium that may be needed.

So called 'adrenal fatigue' is also primarily due to too little salt.

Most people's weight varies randomly across a range equivalent to 2L of water (about 4lbs). A typical 70kg adult contains about 42L of water.

Even an impedance machine will vary with temperature, hydration and emotional stress. Percent body fat is for us a very important metabolic test which should be done by everyone.

**A scale is a lousy tool for monitoring your
HFLC diet – only weigh once a week.**

---

61. SUSTAINING A HIGH FAT LOW CARB DIET

The 'low fat message' published in the media over the last three decades or more is just plain wrong.

Dietary saturated fat has been demonized, whereas published scientific data shows no connection between dietary saturated fat intake and saturated fat levels in the body or any long term risk of heart disease. **There is no need to fear fat.**

In fact, on average the more carbohydrates you eat, the higher the content of saturated fat in the body. Just because you decide to stop eating sugar, bread, potatoes, rice and pasta doesn't mean you have a WFKD for long term use.

It is critical that a HFLC diet must contain an appropriate fat content to be sustainable, safe, and effective.

When you are Keto adapted, fat becomes your body's favorite fuel – carbs must be very low and moderate protein. There is no scientific evidence to support that a moderate protein diet causes kidney disease. When on maintenance, CARB and protein stay pretty consistent, but the amount of fat will change with fat loss.

Contrary to popular belief, a HFLC diet does not lead to muscle loss or impaired physical performance. To maintain a moderate state of nutritional ketosis (1-2mM BOHB) usually requires carb intake of 20-50gm/day and plenty of healthy fat.

For example, one can add 5 tablespoons of olive oil per day on salads, and cook with a diet of meat, poultry, fish, eggs and cheese (80-100gm) and 20gm/total CARBS/day to have great results.

If you don't lose your fear of fat, you can't do a Keto (HFLC) diet.

---

62. KETONES - TO MEASURE OR NOT?

Nutritional Ketosis is defined as a serum ketone ranging from 0.5 to 5 depending on dietary carb and protein consumed. Most people who eat 100gm of carbs and 100gm of protein will drive serum ketones below 0.5mM.

Within a few days on a HFLC diet, the kidneys begin excreting ketones (acetoacetate strips are positive) not BOHB. Betahydroxy butyrate (BOHB) and acetoacetate are made in the liver in equal amounts and both initially are oxidized in muscle. Over a few weeks, the muscles stop using these ketones for fuel.

Instead, muscle cells take up the acetoacetate and reduce it to BOHB and return it into the circulation so that BOHB is the predominant ketone found in the blood which is the preferred ketone for the brain. This process of keto adaption moves fuel from fat to liver to muscle to brain.

Measurements of the third ketone, acetone, is excreted in the breath. Researchers are trying to come up with a measurement device. Most people are able to follow a HFLC diet without measuring ketones and do fine. It is useful in a clinical setting (Four Week Diabetes Cure Program) to measure dietary compliance. As ketones go up, sugar comes down. It is RARE to get hypoglycemia unless intense exercise or on hypoglycemic drugs.

Note: Uric acid often increases in the first week or two of a HFLC diet due to competition of uric acid and ketones for excretion. Within 4-6 weeks this level drops to the same or lower level as part of the body's adaption to nutritional ketosis.

Just because you have ketones doesn't mean you will lose weight. Increased insulin sensitivity and the correct amount of fat will help you lose weight

---

63. SUGAR - TO MEASURE OR NOT?

The Diabetes Control and Complications Trials (DCCT), carried out between 1983-2005, showed that intensive insulin therapy for type I diabetes was worth the risks for the proven cardiovascular benefits, establishing the fact that high glucose levels are toxic to type I diabetes.

This is not the case for type II diabetes treated with insulin. Several studies have confirmed this as mentioned previously. In fact, all standard treatments for type II diabetes including insulin, metformin, SUs and T2Ds had failed to improve health. All trials agreed that intensive glucose control with medications in type II diabetes did not save lives and had marginal, if any, benefits.

The primary reason to measure sugar in type II diabetes is to avoid hypoglycemia from medications. This is especially true when you move from a Standard American Diet to a Ketogenic diet with Intermittent Fasting as you will find a rapid fall in sugar levels. This is where your physician needs to monitor you closely, often during the first 2-3 weeks, as the medications are adjusted or discontinued. Increased on going spikes in sugars, especially after meals, are more worrisome than more stable sugars and increase morbidity.

The newer drugs, SGLT2 inhibitors and Acarbose, do lower both sugar and insulin and should prove to lower end organ damage due to the lower insulin levels.

**A HFLC diet and IF is always the primary
therapy for type II diabetes and obesity.**

64. THE ROLE OF EXERCISE IN DIABESITY

When you gain control of your body, you will gain control of your life. Lack of exercise is a risk factor for more than 25 diseases including type II diabetes and cardiovascular disease. Both resistance and aerobic exercise will benefit type II diabetes but is not as helpful as a HFLC diet and I.F. One of the single most important determinants to cure diabetes is fat loss. Exercise has been shown not to decrease weight. However, meta- analysis shows that exercise may reduce HbA1c without a change in body mass. At least 40 mins, 5 days a week is best.

Resistance training is a potent stimulus to increase muscle mass and strength, and thus there is good reason to consider weight training together with a keto diet for improving body composition, insulin sensitivity, and functional capacity.

- Exercise has been shown to add between 6-7 years to a lifespan and improves the quality of life in countless ways.

- Try to always include a warm-up, flexibility, core/abdominal, balance, cardio and resistance exercise with a cool down period.

- Exercise in the morning or in a fasting state will help you burn more fat and regenerate your mitochondria.

- Exercise improves insulin resistance, increases telomere length, improves your gut microbiome, improves hormones, lowers stress, improves sex drive and mood while preventing cardio-metabolic disease. (It does not produce weight loss)

- More frequent High Intensity Training (HIT) throughout the day is very beneficial to counter-act the prolonged sitting (sitosis) that most of us do all day long.

- Exercise like diet should be intermittent. A Keto Diet is the diet for any athlete!

Adopt a daily exercise routine that best suits you.

65. THE ROLE OF SLEEP IN DIABETES

We are in the midst of a sleep deprivation crisis, with profound consequences to our health, our job performance, our relationships, and our happiness. What we need is nothing short of a sleep revolution: only by renewing our relationship with sleep can we take back control of our lives.

- Arianna Huffington

Sleep duration has been declining over the past decades from the average of nine hours in 1910 to less than six hours for a large number of people today. Sleeping less than 5-6 hours is associated with a 50% increase in weight gain.

Sleep deprivation will stimulate cortisol and decrease insulin sensitivity. In fact, just 24 hours of no sleep will make you insulin resistant. Sleep deprivation can increase the risk of diabetes besides increasing your weight.

Chronic sleep deprivation can also shorten your telomeres (long telomeres are associated with longevity).

- Sleep is far more important for fat loss than exercise.
- Most of us needs 7-8 hours of deep uninterrupted sleep (best to go to bed before 11pm in a dark, cool, quiet room).
- Avoid cellphones, I-pads, computers 2 hours before bedtime (blue light).
- Avoid exercise, excess alcohol, fructose, and heavy meals before bedtime.
- A great cocktail I like for sleep is Vit D3 (5000IU) plus Magnesium Citrate (500mg) and Melatonin (3mg SR) with a mouthful of water when you turn off the light.

**Mobile devices can monitor the quantity
and quality of your sleep.**

66. BALANCE ALL HORMONES NOT JUST INSULIN

Hormones are the juice of life and we age largely because our hormones decline. Although insulin and leptin levels are key in metabolic medicine, there are several other hormones that must be optimized, especially thyroid and sex hormones.

Nearly 50% of 50 year olds have thyroid dysfunction and often testosterone and other sex hormones are depleted and need replacement.

- Hormones are vital to our health. By the time you get to your 40/50's, you are usually on "empty" and need to be "topped up."

- Replace all hormones to the level of a "35 year old" to optimize wellbeing and prevent chronic disease.

- Educate yourself on Menopause and Andropause.

- Beware of blood tests to measure thyroid – they are often wrong and other advanced testing is needed with T3/T4 replacement (not just T4).

- Hormones are essential for mood, weight loss, beauty, sugar control, mitochondrial function, etc.

- Peptides are emerging as a natural safe adjunct to bio-identical hormones.

- Always combine a Keto/Paleo Diet, Exercise and good Sleep that will enhance hormone levels.

- You must keep your 'insulin levels' low to avoid 'insulin resistance' and cardio-metabolic disease that kills 80% of us.

- Measure all your major hormones with a blood, urine or sputum test. (Dutch test best)

Find a physician knowledgeable in Bio-identical (not synthetic) hormones.

---

67. STRESS CAUSES INSULIN RESISTANCE

As mentioned, chronic stress can cause obesity and diabetes; it is no wonder that it has been linked to Alzheimer's disease.

Like insulin, cortisol makes you fat – the stress hormone cortisol enhances glucose availability. In the short term this is good, however under chronic stress glucose levels remain high for months without resolution. Cortisol will increase insulin levels and weight gain. This is the reason that sleep deprivation (high cortisol) helps make people fat. Meditation, yoga, massage and exercise can all help lower cortisol levels.

- People are disturbed not by a thing but by their perception of a thing – the major cause of stress.

- Whatever you do physically has an impact on consciousness, likewise every thought you have registers a physical effect on the body.

- Mindfulness is about waking up, connecting with our deeper selves and appreciating the fullness of each moment of life.

- Meditation is different from mindfulness – all meditation techniques use a comfortable position, a passive attitude, a quite environment, and a "mantra." This is different from mindfulness (emptying the mind) and is known as one pointed-meditation (a 'mantra' stops the mind wandering).

- Mindfulness is paying attention in a particular way, on purpose, in the present moment – and non-judgmentally. It is "the art of conscious living" and is known as Mindfulness Meditation.

- The key to mindfulness is not so much on what you focus on, but the quality of the awareness you bring to each moment – more of a "silent witnessing" or dispassionate observing, than a running commentary on your inner experience.

- Many of the latest scientific findings on Mindfulness come from the Annual Scientific Conference on Mindfulness in Boston each year highlighting its effectiveness for heart disease, stress, blood pressure, mental health, immunity, obesity, diabetes, and aging itself.

- By recognizing and integrating our previous co-present structures of consciousness, we develop "integral consciousness." We become transparent to the transcendent (to the ever present origin).

- Mindfulness is increasingly recognized as an effective way to reduce stress, increase self-awareness, enhance emotional intelligence and effectively handle unpleasant thoughts and feelings and chronic disease.

- Heart Rate Variability (HRV) helps us see the balance of our parasympathetic and sympathetic nervous systems.

Adopt a few simple practices to lower stress and increase mindfulness.

---

68. THE BEST HYPOGLYCEMIC AGENTS

Between 2004 and 2013, no less than 30 new diabetic drugs came to market. Almost 1/3 of diabetics in the US use some form of insulin. None of the newer insulins are better than an older version like Lantus and probably the majority of diabetics are getting little benefit from insulin as mentioned previously.

Oral hypoglycemics are not the answer either and also provide dubious results. Thus, the classic treatment used to treat type II diabetes are questionable as they all don't solve the root cause of diabetes – **our diet.**

Oral Hypoglycemics in type 2 diabetes: A comparison

	Weight Loss	**Weight Neutral**	**Weight Gain**
Drugs	Acarbose SGLT2 inhibitors GLP-1 analogues	Metformin DPP-4 inhibitors	Insulin Sulfonylureas TZDs
Insulin Levels	Lowers Insulin	Neutral	Raises Insulin
Cardiovascular Outcomes compared to metformin	Decreases heart attacks and death	Neutral	Increases heart attacks and death
Verdict?	GOOD	BAD	UGLY

Adapted From Jason Fung MD

A Keto Diet is far more effective for diabetes than any drug.

---

69. A CLOSER LOOK AT ORAL HYPOGLYCEMICS

Sulfonylureas (SUs) and Thiazolidinediones (TZDs) together with insulin all cause weight gain and probably should not be used in type II diabetes.

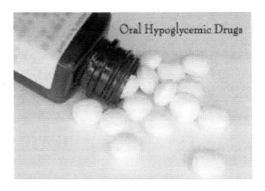
Oral Hypoglycemic Drugs

Metformin and Dipeptidyl peptidase 4 (DPP4) inhibitors do not increase weight although they reduce sugar; they also do not address the root cause of disease (getting rid of sugar is not the same as lowering sugar). Metformin does appear to be safe and may provide some longevity benefits.

Sodium-Glucose cotransporter 2 (SGLT2) inhibitors lower glucose levels by getting rid of the sugar and lower the insulin levels by blocking glucose reabsorption in the kidneys (and they lower risk factors for cardiovascular disease).

Alpha Glucosidase inhibitors (Acarbose) that blocks the digestion of carbohydrates similar to a low-carbohydrate diet and lowers insulin levels with a mild lowering of glucose. It reduces cardiovascular disease by 50% and HT by 34%.

Glucagon-like peptide 1 (GLP1) analogs mimic the effect of incretin hormones which slows down the motility of the stomach and increases satiety. It also lowers cardiovascular risk, but not as well as SGLT2 and Acarbose.

SGLT2, Acarbose and Metformin are my favorites.

---

70. BLOOD PRESSURE AND DIABETES

Most hypertension (high blood pressure) is called "idiopathic hypertension" which means no cause can be found.

Indigenous cultures around the globe tend to maintain their blood pressures reasonably constant throughout their lives. In the West, blood pressure in most of us tends to rise with age.

We have known for 50 years that there is a higher level of insulin in those with hypertension. A complete review of multiple studies done since this time shows that hyperinsulinemia increases the risk of high blood pressure by 63%.

Insulin increases blood pressure through many mechanisms:

1. insulin increases cardiac output.

2. insulin increases sodium reabsorption in the kidneys increasing blood volume

3. insulin stimulates the secretion of anti-diuretic hormone (ADH) increasing blood volume.

4. insulin also increases sympathetic drive centrally

5. insulin constricts blood vessels

6. sugar (high insulin) also causes endothelial dysfunction and stiffening of arteries.

Hypertension is a key marker of metabolic syndrome now affecting 1 in 3 adults in many countries.

Hyperinsulinemia also causes obesity. Hypertension is also seen in PCOS and other cardio-metabolic disease. The root cause of all this disease is excess sugar, grains, and vegetable oils. Weight loss, HFLC diets, and IF are very effective in normalizing blood pressure. Often with Keto diets the blood pressure medication needs to be lowered or stopped.

A Keto Diet and weight loss will often cure hypertension.

71. STATINS AND DIABESITY

The proposed link between blood cholesterol and heart disease was the driving force behind statin therapy. Statins have shown minimal success in reducing cardiovascular disease, and many believe it's statins anti-inflammatory effect that is the mechanism behind this, not the lowering of cholesterol. Dietary therapy to lower saturated fats and LDL-C have not shown any positive effects on lowering heart disease.

The Lyon Diet Heart Study showed that two groups of patients with the same LDL-cholesterol put on a Mediterranean Diet (40% fat) were markedly better off than on an American Heart Association (AHA) (30% low fat) diet in preventing heart disease.

Today we know that LDL-C is a complex mixture of lipoproteins consisting of particles of various sizes. Small LDL particles are much smaller and are very atherogenic (dangerous) while the larger (beach ball) ones are OK. High carb diets consistently and significantly increase the number of small LDL particles, whereas a HFLC diet reduces them.

The LDL-C may increase slightly during the weight loss phase of a HFLC diet, but has no risk of any increased heart disease, as the increase is due to the larger LDL particles.

Cholesterol lowering drugs (statins) have over 142 side effects and dubious benefits, while a HFLC diet has proven benefits that lower the risk of heart disease without any side effects. Statins also increase "insulin resistance."

**A TG/HDL ratio above 2.5 indicates you probably have
pattern B with a predominance of small LDL particles
and a good chance you have insulin resistance.**

---

72. AMPK IN METABOLIC DISEASE AND AGING

Energy balance is maintained by "nutrient sensors" in multiple tissues and organs. Any defect associated with these pathways can lead to cardio-metabolic disease and aging including obesity, diabetes, and metabolic syndrome.

AMPK and MTOR appear to be two of the most important "sensors" and play a significant role in the intermediary metabolism of cardio-metabolic disorders.

AMPK ↑	Fat Burning		AMPK	inflammation
AMPK	insulin sensitivity		AMPK	tumor growth
AMPK	autophagy/ apoptosis		AMPK	oxidative stress (ROS)
AMPK	mitochondrial biogenesis		AMPK	lipogenesis
AMPK	e NOS		AMPK	NFKB
AMPK	FOXO, P53, SIRT1, LKB		AMPK ↓	macrophage, inflammation

FACTORS THAT INCREASE AMPK SIGNALING

GENERAL	NUTRACEUTICALS	HERBS	PHARMACEUTICALS
↓ ATP	Fish Oil	Quercitin	Metformin
↑ AMP	Alpha Lipoic Acid	Berberine	Rapamycin
HFLC Diet	Vitamin C	Artemisinin	Aspirin
↓ Calories	CoQ10	Curcumin	Thyroid (T3)
Youth (age)	Resveratrol	Astralagus	
Cold	Zinc	Hispidulin (snow lotus)	
Black Tea (Theaflavin)	Ginseng (Panax)	Genistein	
Green Tea (EGCG)	Vitamin K2	Gynostemma pentaphyllum	
Rooibos Tea	Fisetin	Trans-tiliroside (rose hips)	
Olive Oil			
Activity (exercise)			
Balanced Deep Sea Water			

AMPK switches away from rapid glycolysis observed in Cancer Cells (Warburg Effect) toward oxidative metabolism found in mitochondria of normal cells.

---

73. MTOR IN METABOLIC DISEASE AND AGING

MTOR (mammalian target of rapamycin) Rapamycin, found in the soil of Easter Island in 1965, was made by bacteria to target yeast. MTOR in some sense is the secret for how life is organized within the cell and operates in close communication with the nucleus of all cells. MTORs primary purpose is growth and development. Rapamycin can be used for extension of healthy lifespan and prevention of age-related diseases like obesity, diabetes, and metabolic syndrome by slowing down the aging process.

Both by ↓ MTOR and ↑ AMPK you can extend the human lifespan.

MTOR ↑ protein synthesis
MTOR | cell growth
MTOR | hyperfunction (cells)

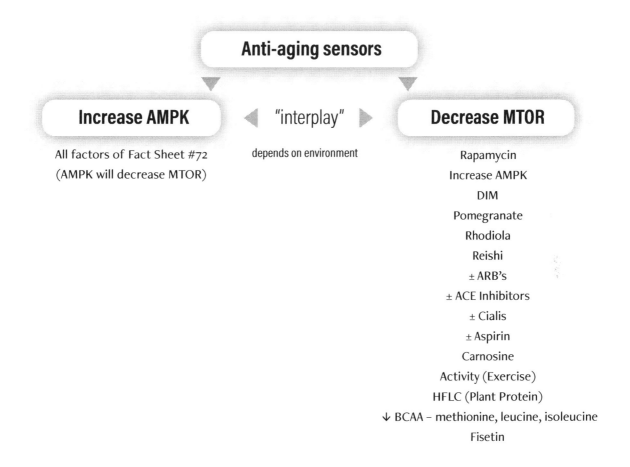

Anti-aging sensors

Increase AMPK | ◀ "interplay" ▶ | Decrease MTOR

Increase AMPK	depends on environment	Decrease MTOR
All factors of Fact Sheet #72 (AMPK will decrease MTOR)		Rapamycin
		Increase AMPK
		DIM
		Pomegranate
		Rhodiola
		Reishi
		± ARB's
		± ACE Inhibitors
		± Cialis
		± Aspirin
		Carnosine
		Activity (Exercise)
		HFLC (Plant Protein)
		↓ BCAA – methionine, leucine, isoleucine
		Fisetin

Rapamycin can be characterized as calorie restriction (up to 40%) in a pill. It can be used off label in smaller weekly doses under the supervision of a physician. It has been found helpful in obesity, diabetes, metabolic syndrome, cardio-metabolic disease, and aging.

---

74. NUTRACEUTICALS AND DIABETES

Nutraceuticals can be broadly defined as components of foods or dietary supplements that have a medicinal or therapeutic effect. In general, nutraceuticals are taken in higher amounts than that which can be obtained from a regular diet.

We have formulated the Magnificent 7 with berberine, gynostemma, quercetin, epicatechin, vit. C, resveratrol, and alpha-lipoic acid- all AMPK stimulants that will lower sugar and insulin and increase mitochondrial biogenesis. Other core nutraceuticals need to be part of a comprehensive approach to reverse diabesity.

- Nearly all disease develops at the cellular level (40 trillion cells) within our different organs usually associated with inflammation.

- Cardiovascular and Neurological disease are most common as these two organs consume nutraceuticals at higher rates than other organs.

- Vital nutrients are needed for the thousands of biochemical reactions going on in each cell to minimize inflammation and telomere shortening.

- The primary cause of cellular malfunction is a deficiency in 1 or more vital nutrients – vitamins, minerals, hormones and other essential nutrients.

- Metabolic and psychological stress will change the demand for nutrients needed by the various cells and organs.

- Nutrients are required in different amounts depending on genetic disposition, age, lifestyle, medical history, pollution, and biochemical individuality.

- Today, all people need to supplement their diet due to the degradation of the soil, air and water and farming practices especially those with Diabesity.

- **Core Nutraceuticals** should be taken by everyone - Vit D3, Magnesium, Omega 3's, Magnificent 7, Telovite (multivitamin).

- **Targeted Nutraceuticals** are used as natural therapy targeting specific organs to optimize their function when hyperinsulinemia has damaged them.

- You should have all your vitamins, minerals, fatty acids, enzymes, anti-oxidants, amino acids measured with a simple blood test.

It is essential to take Core Nutraceuticals daily.

---

75. CORE NUTRACEUTICALS FOR DIABETES

1. **Magnificent 7:** We have mentioned the 7 active ingredients that enhance AMPK and help reverse diabesity.

2. **Omega 3-FA:** Only two good sources, fish and brains of animals (No good plant sources), need both EPA and DHA. Decreases heart disease, abnormal heart rhythm, sudden death. Also decreases risk of cancer, autoimmune disease, cognitive disease, and lowers blood pressure and triglycerides.

3. **Telovit-Multivitamin:** Due to current Agri Business and Big Food, it is worth taking a multivitamin to ensure adequate nutrition. Telovite multivitamins was the first multivitamin proven by us to extend telomeres that enhance longevity.

4. **Magnesium:** Those who have diabesity have low magnesium levels. Magnesium decreases blood sugar, blood pressure, and abnormal heart rhythms. It can also decrease migraines and muscle cramps. Also helps constipation and osteoporosis.

5. **Vitamin D3:** More than 90% of people, especially diabetics, have low D3 levels. A normal range is 70-80 (not 30-50). Vit D3 decreases inflammation throughout the body and boosts immunity. Vit D3 lowers risk for heart disease, cancer, diabetes, depression, osteoporosis and autoimmune disease.

6. **CoQ10:** Is a powerful antioxidant and improves mitochondrial function. Helps correct abnormal heart rhythms and intractable heart failure. It helps lower blood pressure and reduces clotting of blood. Produces increased energy in all cells in the body.

7. **Vit K2:** Protects bones, diabetes, cancer and prevents arteries from calcification. People with the highest levels of vitamin K2 are 36% less likely to die from all causes – i.e. it extends lifespan.

8. **Iodine:** Many people have subclinical hypothyroidism that makes it difficult to lose weight. Iodine decreases cysts in thyroid, breast and ovaries and lowers risk of cancer. It is also good for oral health and will often itself correct hypothyroidism.

9. **Methylfolate and Methylcobalamin:** Half of the globe has one or more mutations of the methylenetetrahydrofolate reductase (MTHFR) gene – the "Mother F'er" gene which limits their ability to make the active forms of folate and B12 raising homocysteine levels.

Most of us need several core nutraceuticals.

---

76. LECTINS, LPS AND LEAKY GUT

My colleague, Dr. Steven Gundry, has recognized a **KEY** problem underlying most of the disease of civilization (cardio-metabolic disease) like diabetes, heart disease, cancer, Alzheimer's, Parkinson's, etc. This problem is the breakdown of the intestinal barrier (leaky gut) due to **lectins** and the deadly gut disruptors: antibiotics, antacids, NSAIDs, artificial sweeteners, endocrine disruptors, GMO foods, pesticides, blue light, and the HCLF diet.

Lipopolysaccharides (LPS) are molecules that make up the cell walls of certain bacteria in our microbiome- "little pieces of shit" that travel through your gut wall into your body. Your body treats these molecules as a threat and summons your white blood cells for an attack causing inflammation. The "lectins" bear a similarity to many of our important organs, nerves and joints – through this "molecular mimicry" and depending on your genetics confuses the body's messaging and produces auto-immunity (friendly fire).

More importantly, lectins and LPS cause mitochondrial dysfunction. Mitochondria produce our energy by using sugar and fats to produce ATP in the Krebs cycle. Ketones are generated from fat cells when sugar supplies are low (night, winter, fasting). Due to our modern lifestyles and abundance of HCLF diets and constant light, our mitochondria work overtime. (It takes half of the energy to turn ketones (HFLC) into ATP than it does with sugar.) When your mitochondria are under this stress, your energy levels plummet and you develop "insulin resistance" (See #40-45) which is how lectins and LPS help cause obesity and autoimmune diseases like diabetes.

Protein can be as big a problem as sugar and carbohydrates which is why many on the Keto diet fail to maintain Ketosis as they take their good fat, but too generous amounts of animal protein like bacon, spare ribs, beef, sausages, cold cuts, as well as high-fat cheeses.

Several plant fats are composed of Ketones. MCT oils are 100% ketones, solid coconut oil contains 65% ketones, palm fruit oil has 50% ketones, butter and ghee have butyrate and may provide better choices.

If you have diabetes or other autoimmune disease, avoid lectins.

---

77. INFLAMMATION AND DIABETES

As early as the 1950's, there was evidence to show a correlation between inflammation and insulin resistance states like obesity and diabetes.

Obesity-induced chronic inflammation is a key component causing insulin resistance and metabolic syndrome. Pro-inflammatory cytokines can cause insulin resistance in adipose tissue, skeletal muscle, and the liver. Inflammation in the gut can also cause insulin and leptin resistance.

There is a strong interconnection between obesity, inflammation, and insulin resistance. People with other inflammatory disease are at higher risk for type II diabetes. (IL10 is an anti-inflammatory cytokine produced by macrophages. There is a greater incidence of insulin resistance in people with reduced levels of IL10).

- Research shows that all chronic disease has a significant inflammatory component and you need to know how to control it.

- Silent inflammation attacks the single layer of cells – the endothelium – that line the 50,000 miles of blood vessels within each of us, hence its widespread effects.

- The major cause of silent inflammation is the result of the changes that have occurred in our food supply over the past 50 years. The increase in sugar, grains, and plant oils are the main problems in our modern diet.

- A Paleo Diet (mod carb, mod protein, mod fat) or Keto Diet (low carb, mod protein, high fat) are the best ways to lower inflammation.

- In addition to controlling the metabolic stress (insulin resistance) with diet, you also need to control psychological stress which is the other primary cause of cellular inflam-aging and telomere shortening.

- Lectins (gluten is the most common lectin known) are found in many grains, fruits and vegetables, e.g. Nightshades can cause low grade inflammation throughout the body. Anyone with autoimmune disease should avoid lectins. (See Plant Paradox by Steven Gundry MD) – this includes diabetics.

- Avoid all toxins – personal care products, EMF, insecticides, GMO foods, stress, heavy metals, cigarettes, drugs, polluted water, and air.

- Select Nutraceuticals like turmeric, fish oil, anti-oxidants, quercitin, vitamin C, bergamet, magnificent 7 and metformin should be taken regularly.

- It is important to pay attention to **all** of the root-causes of disease and balance all key I.N.T.E.G.R.A.L. Health components!

You can measure simple blood markers for inflammation like ESR, C-reactive protein, IL1, IL6, IL8, TNF, homocysteine, etc.

---

78. DIABETES AND THE GUT MICROBIOME

There are at least 100 times more genes in the human microbiome than in the human genome. Recently the potential role of the gut microbiome in obesity and diabetes has been recognized.

A healthy biome is characterized by bacterial diversity and richness. Gut microbiota are mostly comprised of Firmicutes (64%), Bacteroidetes (23%), Proteobacteria (8%), and Actinobacteria (3%).

Those on a HFLC diet have a Bacteroides dominant pattern. Those on a HCLF diet have a Provotella dominant pattern, lack of bacterial diversity and overgrowth of pathobacteria resulting in dysbiosis, an imbalance in the ecology of the gut. Dysbiosis is correlated with obesity, diabetes, as well as other autoimmune diseases.

The microbiome of **type II diabetics** have increased Bacteroidetes/Firmicutes ratio that correlates with plasma glucose levels.

The microbiome of some **obese** patients have decreased Bacteroidetes/ Firmicutes ratio compared to type II diabetes.

Patients with type II diabetes have decreased amounts of butyrate producing bacteria. Butyrate acetate (Ketones) are fermented in the large intestine from dietary fiber. Butyrate maintains intestinal integrity (energy in) that prevents gram negative intestinal bacteria **LPS** from crossing the gut wall preventing endotoxemia.

Endotoxemia triggers a low grade inflammatory response and low grade inflammation thought to underlie type II diabetes and other cardio-metabolic disease.

Therapeutic intervention like HFLC diets, prebiotics, probiotics, metformin, fecal transplantation and Bariatric surgery can effectively alter the composition of gut bacteria.

Most prebiotics are oligosaccharides, e.g. asparagus, garlic, onions and wheat bran. Pickled and fermented foods are good sources of both prebiotics and probiotics.

- Avoid all antibiotics
- Avoid artificial sweeteners
- Avoid OTC eg. NSAIDS
- Beware Lectin Foods
- Eat insoluble fiber
- Eat fermented foods
- Avoid blue light
- At least 7 hours sleep
- Avoid stress
- Avoid pesticides

Take a "Selfie" of your microbiome with a Q-tip of stool.

---

79. TOXIC HEAVY METALS AND DIABETES

Heavy metals like arsenic, zinc, cadmium, mercury, lead, and nickel have all been associated with damage to the mitochondria including the islet cells of the pancreas and increased risk of type II diabetes.

Uncontrolled industrialization has produced this heavy metal pollution in the world.

Cigarette smoke is a primary source of cadmium and should be avoided for the damage it can cause to the pancreas as well as its risk for cardio-metabolic disease in diabetes.

- The WHO estimates that within the next decade cancer will surpass cardiac disease as the #1 killer and 1:3 people will develop cancer.

- Cancer is also a 'metabolic disease.' Faulty nutrition and an increasing toxic load has lead to this man-made disease by damaging the mitochondria in your body. Heavy metals are very damaging to the mitochondria.

- Otto Warburg, MD showed in the 1930's that sugar is the main nutrient for cancer cells (Obesity increases risk of cancer 10x). Avoid animal protein in cancer.

- The CDC estimates that 25% of the US population alone are toxic with heavy metals which also increases the risk of obesity, diabesity, and cancer.

- Identify all toxins in your home, work place, and neighborhood environment.

- Beware of all electromagnetic devices, phones, computers, microwaves, etc. and buy organic foods whenever possible.

- Select supplements – alpha lipoic acid, milk-thistle, chelating agents, etc. that can all help to detoxify you.

- Employ regular detoxification rituals – fasting, colon therapy, regular exercise, Far Infra-Red (FIR) Saunas etc.

- Cancer, like Diabetes, Heart Diseases and Alzheimer's has a long prodromal period and this is why simple screening is necessary to diagnose mutations in the prodromal stage.

- Two tests I recommend are a simple urine test to detect heavy metals and a yearly 'liquid biopsy' once you are over the age of 35-40 years to screen for cancer. (See Bioscience)

Beware of heavy metals and mitochondrial dysfunction.

---

80. THE KETOGENIC DIET PROTECTS OUR MITOCHONDRIA

Energy sources from fat don't require processing (like sugar) and go directly to the mitochondria to provide energy. In fact, both the brain and heart run more efficiently on Ketones than sugar.

In addition to the energy they produce, mitochondria also produce a byproduct from oxidation called reactive oxygen species (ROS) known as free radicals. When we burn fuel from fat, we not only get more energy (48 ATP) as compared to CARBS (36 ATP), but we produce ketones that decrease oxidative stress that prevents over excitation of the cell.

This process is especially important for the mitochondria's own DNA (referred to as mtDNA) which is separate from the DNA in the nucleus (n-DNA), as mtDNA is especially vulnerable to free radical damage as it lacks a protective protein coat (histones). If we don't consume enough fat, we can't build a functional mitochondrial membrane which will keep them healthy and prevent them from dying. Cells in our brain, muscles, heart, kidney and liver contain thousands of mitochondria comprising up to 40% of the cells mass. According to Professor Enzo Nisoli, a human adult possesses more than 10 million billion mitochondria making up a full 10% of the total body weight.

- Eat a Keto Diet free of processed and GMO foods.
- Avoid all broad spectrum antibiotics.
- Avoid all OTC drugs like antacids, non-steroidal inflammatory drugs etc.
- Avoid all artificial sweeteners and sodas.
- Beware all "lectin" containing foods. (#82)
- Get at least 7 hours sleep each night.
- Eat fermented foods and plenty of insoluble fiber.
- Avoid constant stress and blue light exposure.
- Take prebiotics and probiotics.
- Take a 'selfie' of your microbiome (gut bugs) with a simple Q-tip of stool – vital for your wellbeing.

The Keto Diet reduces dysfunction of Mitochondria and enhances mitochondrial biogenesis. Ketones produce more energy (48 ATP) than glucose (36 ATP) at less cost.

---

81. LECTINS INCREASE RISK OF DIABETES AND OBESITY

Many plant-based foods, such as beans, legumes, fruits, vegetables and whole grains contain high amounts of lectins (see #82). Lectins can impact health in multiple ways from digestion and skin rashes to serious chronic diseases. Cooking methods that use moist heat are helpful to reduce the amounts of lectins (Dry heat also increases AGE's).

Gluten (perhaps the best known lectin) is often blamed for being the sole source of wheat problems, but it is really gliadin, a smaller protein within gluten, that does most of the damage. If you eat an egg, the protein is degraded into single amino acids. Not so with gliadin, it is broken down into 'peptides' (short chains of amino acids). These peptides enter the blood stream and go to the same receptors as heroin and morphine with multiple neurological symptoms. Even more harmful is their addictive quality and their ability to stimulate appetite – demonstrating consistent increases in calorie intake to the tune of 400 cals per day. Not only wheat, but rye and barley are also potent appetite stimulants with other mind-altering effects.

Beware of the "so called gluten-free products" which are actually full of lectins in the form of flour made from corn, oats, buckwheat, quinoa and pseudo-grains, as well as soy-beans and other legumes. Many of these products will increase your weight. They also have transglutaminase which can cross the blood brain barrier and disrupt neurotransmitters.

Similarly, "whole grain" foods are just as unhealthy and often much higher in lectins. Asians have stripped the hull of brown rice to make it white before they eat it, i.e. white rice (and white bread) which are a lot easier on the gut.

The NLRP3 inflammasome (inflammasome are assembled in response to certain "danger signals" in the body) is responsible for the release of pro-inflammatory cytokines, such as IL-1B and IL-18, and is probably responsible for the pathogenesis of various inflammatory diseases including diabetes, obesity, cardiovascular, Alzheimer's, autoimmune disease, gout, arthritis, among others.

Food intolerances and allergies lead to chronic digestive and autoimmune disease. One of the key factors are lectins from grains, legumes, and dairy. Lectins can bind to numerous carbohydrate containing receptors on cell surfaces. Endoplasmic stress triggers mitochondrial dysfunction and inflammasome activation through NLRP3. This causes secretion of pro-inflammatory cytokines causing chronic inflammation central to all chronic cardio-metabolic disease.

Consider going on a Keto-Lectin Free Diet.

---

82. LECTIN FOODS TO AVOID

THE JUST SAY "NO" LIST OF LECTIN-CONTAINING FOOD

Non-Southern European Cow's Milk Products (these contain casein A-1)
- Yogurt
- Greek Yogurt
- Ice cream
- Frozen yogurts
- Cheese
- Ricotta
- Cottage cheese
- Kefir
- Casein protein powders

Grains-or Soybean-Fed Fish, Shellfish, Poultry, Beef, Lamb and Pork

Sprouted Grains, Psuedo-Grains, Grasses
Whole Grains
- Wheat (pressure cooking does not remove lectins from any form of wheat)
- Einkorn wheat
- Kamut
- Oats (cannot pressure cook)
- Quinoa
- Rye (cannot pressure cook)
- Bulgur
- Brown Rice
- White Rice
- Wild Rice

Fruits (some we call vegetables)
All fruits, including berries
Cucumbers
- Zucchini
- Pumpkins
- Squashes (any kind)

- Melons (any kind)
- Eggplant
- Tomatoes
- Bell peppers
- Chili peppers
- Goji berries
- Barley (cannot pressure cook)
- Buckwheat
- Kashi
- Spelt
- Corn
- Corn Products
- Cornstarch
- Corn syrup
- Popcorn
- Wheatgrass
- Barley grass

Oils
- Soy
- Grape seed
- Corn
- Peanut
- Cottonseed
- Safflower
- Sunflower
- "Partially hydrogenated"
- Vegetable
- Canola

Refined, Starchy Foods
- Pasta
- Rice
- Potatoes
- Potato chips
- Milk
- Bread
- Tortillas (except for the two Siete products above)

- Pastry
- Flours made from grains and pseudo-grains
- Cookies
- Crackers
- Cereal
- Sugar
- Agave
- Splenda (sucralose)
- SweetOne or Sunett (acesulfame K)
- NutraSweet (aspartame)
- Sweet'n Low (saccharin)
- Diet drinks
- Maltodextrin

Vegetables
- Peas
- Sugar snap peas
- Legumes
- Green beans
- Chickpeas (including as hummus)
- Soy
- Tofu
- Edamame
- Soy protein
- Textured vegetable protein (TVP)
- All beans, including sprouts
- All lentils

Nuts and Seeds
- Pumpkin
- Sunflower
- Chia
- Peanuts
- Cashews

Adapted from the Plant Paradox by Steven Gundry MD

Author's Note: If you have any Autoimmune Disease like type II diabetes or severe cardio-metabolic disease, I would avoid the "lectin" containing food listed above. It remains to be seen if the rest of us should also avoid these foods!

---

83. DIABETES AND CARDIOVASCULAR DISEASE

Most diabetics die of cardiovascular disease. Cardiac deaths are the leading cause of death, not only in the USA but in most developed countries, of which diabetes is the number one cause. As Dr. Kraft said, "those with cardiovascular disease not identified with diabetes are simply undiagnosed."

Dr. Stout, in 1977, identified the origin of the pathology of type II diabetes as vascular (arterial), directly related to hyperinsulinemia and not to hyperglycemia. The pathology of type II diabetes as outlined is mainly the following:

1. Cardiovascular disease
    a. Coronary artery disease
    b. Congestive heart failure
    c. Idiopathic cardiomyopathy
    d. Coronary microvascular dysfunction
2. Cerebral vascular disease
    a. Stroke – kills over 160,000 a year in the US and often without warning
    b. Transient ischemic attack (TIA)
3. Nephropathy
    a. Hypertension
    b. Nephrosclerosis – arterial and arteriolar
4. Retinopathy – major cause of blindness among adults aged 20-74 years
5. Neuropathy
6. Autonomic – cardiovascular
    a. Peripheral – distal symmetric polyneuritis
    b. Central – neurotological (tinnitus)
    c. Peripheral arterial disease
7. Penile erectile dysfunction
8. Gestational Diabetes
9. Peyronie's Disease, penile arteriosclerosis of the corpora cavernosa with erectile curvature

---

Hyperinsulinemia Not Hyperglycemia Kills!
I, like Joseph Kraft, MD and others, believe 100% of cardiovascular disease is due to "insulin resistance."

---

84. DIABETES AND CANCER

"Most genetic defects found in cancer are 'red herrings' that have diverted attention away from mitochondrial respiratory insufficiency, the central feature of the disease." as Dr. Thomas Seyfried describes in his excellent book: "Cancer is a Metabolic Disease."

- Cancer is a modern day man made epidemic, like obesity and diabetes, caused by faulty dietary practices and an increasing toxic environment.

- Diabetes, as well as obesity and prediabetes, increases the risk of many different types of cancer, including breast, colon, endometrial, ovarian, kidney and bladder cancers.

- Dr. Thomas Seyfried believes that cancer is a metabolic disease. Cancer cells are highly metabolically active and use glucose as their primary fuel. Insulin use increases the risk of cancer at least 20%, and a recent review of newly diagnosed diabetics in a Saskatchewan population showed that the use of insulin raised the risk of cancer 90%.

- Unlike normal cells, the mitochondria in cancer cells are unable to use ketones to generate ATP. Instead, cancer cells rely on the extremely inefficient system of fermentation. This means the average cancer cell needs up to 18x more sugar to grow and divide than normal cells. In addition, cancer cells prefer fructose to ferment.

- Dr. Fung points out that the relationship between cancer and insulin is reinforced by the discovery that a single mutation in the PTEN oncogene significantly raises the risk of breast cancer. In a similar fashion, medications that increase insulin are associated with a higher cancer risk.

By using nutritional ketosis and raising AMPK and decreasing MTOR, the two key metabolic switches, you lower the sugar inside the mitochondria and shift the sugar burning to fat burning which enhances mitochondrial function that lowers inflammation and stabilizes the genome. Cancer cells are weakened and more easily destroyed with lower doses of targeted chemotherapy.

Insulin facilitates every step along the inflammatory pathway that marks the progression of the disease. Treatment with insulin does not lower disease risk, rather, it more than doubles the risk of death as 'hyperinsulinemia' is the cause of all cardio-metabolic disease. The longer the treatment time with insulin and the higher dose, the earlier you die! The solution is a well formulated keto diet and addressing all other lifestyle factors that lower the risk of cancer.

Bioscience does a yearly "liquid biopsy" as part of our Primordial Cancer Prevention program focused on lowering inflammation and increasing genomic stability before a cancer can develop.

---

85. DIABETES AND ALZHEIMER'S

Alzheimer's disease is a chronic, progressive, neurodegenerative disease that causes memory loss, personality changes and dementia. It is the 6th leading cause of death in the USA.

The link between Diabetes and Alzheimer's is so strong that many researchers are calling Alzheimer's "Type III Diabetes."

A longitudinal study in Diabetologia (2018) followed 5,189 people and showed that people with a higher blood sugar had a faster rate of cognitive decline than those with normal sugar.

Currently dementia is not curable, which makes it very important to look for the root-cause.

Professor Melissa Schilling, in 2016, sought to reconcile two confusing trends. People who have type II diabetes are twice as likely to get Alzheimer's, and type I diabetics treated with insulin are also more likely to get Alzheimer's. This shows that elevated insulin is involved. Schilling points out that even in prediabetics, dementia can occur probably due to the hyperinsulinemia (Again often neuroscientists are focused on glucotoxicity rather than on hyperinsulinemia similar to cardiovascular disease).

In 2012, Rosebud Roberts, a professor at Mayo Clinic, broke down 1,000 people into 4 group based on how much carbohydrate they ate. The group that ate the most carbs had an 80% higher chance of having cognitive impairment. There are several possible causes of the relationship between diabetes and dementia:

- Diabetes weakens blood vessels which increase the risk of "mini" strokes.
- Brain cells can become insulin resistant.
- Obesity produces cytokines that cause inflammatory proteins and increase risk
- Obesity doubles the chance of a person's risk of having high amyloid levels

It is important to note, as Daniel Amen, MD points out, that a SPECT scan can diagnose Alzheimer's 30 years before onset of clinical picture. We know that ketones have powerful and lasting epigenetic effects on the brain, even helping reduce the risk of dementia in the APO4 genotype. Also HFLC diets can decrease insulin resistance and lead to autophagy and apoptosis.

A Keto-Diet and I.F. can prevent and help dementia.

---

86. DIABETES AND INFECTIONS

Diabetics are prone to all types of infections. Not only are they more susceptible, but more often the infections are far more serious increasing morbidity and mortality.

The reason for these more frequent infections include:

- Hyperglycemic environment
- Decreased antioxidant system
- Micro and macro vascular disease
- Neuropathy
- GUT and urinary dysmotility
- More medical interventions
- Increase psychological stress

The most common infections include:

1. Respiratory infections – pneumonia, influenza, TB, bronchitis
2. Urinary infections – bladder, kidney, urethra (fungal and bacterial)
3. Gastrointestinal – gastritis, candidiasis, cholecystitis
4. Liver – hepatitis C, hepatitis B
5. Skin – nails, fasciitis, gangrene
6. Head and Neck – sinusitis, rhinitis, periodontitis
7. HIV

Infectious disease may result in more severe metabolic disorders. Despite good blood glucose control, 15% of diabetics will develop non-healing leg wounds and a 15-fold increase in lower limb amputations. Stem cells from adipose tissue from the patient have been shown to produce dramatic shorter wound healing and looks to be cost effective and prevents serious complications.

Be vigilant for any signs of infection.

---

87. DIABETES AND ERECTILE DYSFUNCTION

Diabetes is the most frequent cause of Erectile Dysfunction (ED) increasing the risk more than 3-4 times the average. In some countries like the Middle East and India, ED can affect 50% of men over the age of 40.

The reason for this is poor blood flow and nerve damage. The risk increases with age and severity with the incidence rising to more than 60% with men over the age of 50. Up to 75% of men with diabetes will have some degree of erectile dysfunction.

Erectile dysfunction (impotence) is the inability to maintain an erection firm enough for sex. Half the men with type II diabetes within 5-10 years of their diagnosis will develop ED.

Although lowering risk factors like better control of your sugar, decreasing alcohol intake, exercise, more sleep, and keeping your stress levels down can all help, the key is lowering insulinemia – "insulin resistance"- with a high fat low carb diet and intermittent fasting.

In my experience more than 90% of ED can be treated successfully; hormonal replacement, Cialis, Viagra, Levitra, nutraceuticals, pharmaceuticals, injections of prostaglandins, Gains Wave, implants and pumps can all be used. Treatment needs to be tailored to the individual and depends on the severity of the disease. It is also important to look at cardiac risk factors, as often ED occurs 4-5 years before a cardiac event.

If you have ED, have your heart checked.

---

88. DIABETES AND PCOS

Women with Polycystic ovarian disease (PCOS) are characterized by no periods or irregular periods, increased testosterone, acne and hirsutism and may have cysts on their ovaries and acanthosis nigricans. PCOs patients share many of the same signs as obese diabetic patients – waist size greater than 35", obesity, high blood pressure, abnormal lipid profile and insulin resistance.

PCOS is the most common cause of infertility; eggs have trouble being released from the ovary. Women with diabetes are at increased risk for PCOS. The underlying pathophysiology appears to be "insulin resistance" so that the single best therapy is a HFLC diet and intermittent fasting. Bioidentical hormones and pharmaceuticals that increase insulin sensitivity can also be useful.

PCOS also puts women at increased risk for a variety of more serious diseases like:
1. Obesity
2. Diabetes
3. Heart disease
4. Cancer
5. Hypertension
6. Stroke
7. Depression
8. Metabolic Syndrome
9. Sleep apnea

If you have PCOS and want to get pregnant, go Keto.

89. SKIN MANIFESTATIONS OF DIABETES

Diabetes is an autoimmune disease and you need to be aware that skin disease from insulin resistance or the gut could be the first signs of diabetes.

Metabolic Causes (IR)

1. Bullous Diabeticorum
2. Acanthosis Nigricans
3. Diabetic Dermopathy
4. Necrobiosis Lipoidica Diabeticorum (NLD)
5. Gouty Tophi
6. Hirsuitism
7. Alopecia
8. Seborrhea
9. Acne
10. Foot Ulcer

Autoimmune Causes (Gut)

1. Scleroderma
2. Psoriasis
3. Dermatomyositis
4. Bullous Pemphigoid
5. Pemphigus
6. Lichen Planus
7. Lupus
8. Vasculitis
9. Behcet's Disease
10. Dermatatis Herpetiformis
11. Inflammatory Bowel Disease (Aphthous ulcers, erythema nodosum)
12. Alopecia Areata
13. Pernicious Anemia
14. Thyroid Disease eg. Myxedema
15. Calcinosis (CREST)
16. Discoid Lupus
17. Rosaccea

Skin Disease can alert you to underlying "Insulin Resistance" and autoimmune disease.

---

90. DIABETES AND KIDNEY DISEASE

Although most of the fructose goes to the liver, 30% of fructose goes to the kidney where it directly damages the filtering system.

Excess protein, carbs, and fruit are your enemy. Fat and Ketones are your friends. In fact, fructose is the leading cause of kidney failure – it is toxic candy!

We could tolerate its toxicity for a few months in by gone times, but now our kidneys receive 365 days of direct insult with no breaks. A high fat low carb diet will reverse your diabetes and kidney disease.

Steve Gundry gives a good example in the "Plant Paradox" of how Ketones can help the kidney:

> *"The best example of ketosis in action is a pregnant hibernating bear. She enters her den pregnant but doesn't eat or drink for five months. During that time, she gestates her young, gives birth, suckles her cubs, and emerges from the den skinny but with all her muscle mass intact. If she didn't spare her muscles, she couldn't hunt for food for her cubs. But the most amazing feat of all is that she doesn't urinate for five months. How does she do all this? She lives on the ketones from the fat that she stored for the winner. Now, kidneys have really only two jobs to do: get rid of water that you drink or consume in foods, and filter out protein waste by-products. Like diesel fuel, protein burns dirty; ketones, on the other hand, burn clean, like natural gas. Mama bear burns ketones and drinks nothing, so her kidneys have nothing to do, and therefore she has nothing to urinate."*

**Check your Creatinine, Cystatin C
Level and GFR Kidney Tests.**

---

91. DIABETES AND AUTOIMMUNE DISEASE

The first mistake in our nutrition occurred over 10,000 years ago (just 300 generations ago) in our 2.5 million year history, when we began growing grains (the seeds of grass).

Long before humans (450 million years ago), plants protected themselves from predators by producing toxins, including lectins, in the plant and its seeds.

Lectins are found in almost all plants and other foods in our diet including meat, poultry, and fish.

As Gundry notes: the reason wheat became the grain of choice in northern climates was due to a small lectin known as wheat germ agglutinin (WGA) which is responsible for wheat's weight-gaining propensity (WGA resembles insulin). WGA is also found in barley, rye, and rice and is very toxic to our gut (WGA alone can cause celiac disease).

Wheat, rye, and other grains are also high in fructans. The gut bacteria can convert the fructans to fructose in the gut which can turn on the fat switch and also increase weight.

When cows and other animals eat grains (or soy), these proteins land up in the animal's meat or milk. The same happens in chicken and farm-raised sea foods. Knowing how the food you eat was grown and raised also directly affects your health, as does the way you cook your food.

ORGAN	DISEASE
Gut	Crohn's Disease
Myelin Sheath	Multiple Sclerosis
Pancreas	Diabetes
Joints	Rheumatoid Arthritis
Thyroid	Hashimoto's or Graves
Skin	Psoriasis

Eating refined grains thus not only promotes pathological bugs in our gut, but also the immunogenic properties of some foods (depending also on a person's genetics) which can damage the lining of the gut causing it to become "leaky" which sets the stage for auto-immune disease:

Don't eat grains – wheat, rye, barley, oats, corn, rice, sorghum and millet. Avoid pseudograins – buckwheat, amaranth and quinoa.

---

92. THE ROLE OF FIBER IN DIABETES

People who eat more than 30gms of fiber per day have a 20% lower risk of diabetes. Fiber can change hormonal signals, slow down nutrient absorption, alter fermentation, promote feelings of satiety, and cause weight loss. Fiber is in fact an anti-nutrient and acts as an antidote to excess carbs.

Fiber improves blood sugar by decreasing insulin peaks after a meal and by increasing insulin sensitivity.

Soluble fiber like that in berries, nuts, and some vegetables dissolve into a gel- like substance and helps slow down digestion. Soluble fiber reduces glucose and insulin levels.

Insoluble fiber found in foods like dark green leafy vegetables, celery, and carrots do not dissolve at all and add bulk to your stool.

Certain fibers are prebiotics which can help nourish beneficial bacteria in your gut that enhance digestion and immune function like onions, leeks, and garlic and helps type II diabetes.

Each 10gram increase in fiber intake is associated with a 15% lower mortality from all causes; e.g. for every 10gm increase of fiber consumed, the chance of stroke decreases by 10%.

Fiber can protect against insulin and thus prevent type II diabetes as was shown in the Nurses' Health Study. Nurses who ate the highest glycemic diet but also ate the highest fiber diet had no increase in diabetes.

Top 10 Foods with Fiber (Lectin Free)

1. Green Plantains
2. Green Bananas
3. Celery Root
4. Glucomannan (Konjac root)
5. Green Papaya
6. Cauliflower
7. Brussel Sprouts
8. Root Vegetables – onions, sweet potatoes
9. Sorghum
10. Millet

A simple rule is to get most of your fiber in the form of vegetables, nuts (not cashews or peanuts) and seeds (not chia, pumpkin and sunflower seeds). Avoid all grains, fruit, and all processed foods.

---

4 Week Diabetis Cure · Graham Simpson MD

93. DRINKS FOR KETO DIETS

Start your day with a Bullet Proof Coffee or Chai Tea

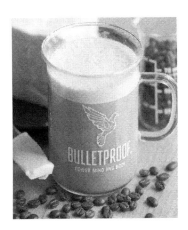

The Bullet-Proof Diet, written by Dave Asprey, is a dietary approach for rapid weight loss and better cognitive health. It recommends getting 50-70% of your energy from healthy fats, especially MCT oil, grass fed butter, and coconut oil. The plan's 'signature breakfast' is "bullet proof coffee" (a mix of coffee, MCT oil and butter). It decreases hunger levels, provides the ability to fast easily, and enhances better brain function and clarity. You can use coconut butter instead of coconut oil or MCT oil. Coconut butter is made from the entire flesh of the coconut that is ground to create a creamy paste. Coconut and MCT oil use solvents and heat to extract pure fatty acids while the flesh is discarded. If you prefer tea over coffee, you add butter or coconut oil in the same way.

BULLETPROOF COFFEE

1. Coffee Beans (less moldy-preferably Arabica for example)
2. Grassfed Butter (Kerrygold butter) or Grassfed Ghee
3. Organic Virgin Coconut oil (Clearspring Organic Virgin Coconut Oil, Organic Langer) You can use coconut butter, coconut oil or MCTs
4. Cinnamon or Vanilla for taste

How to make a delicious Bulletproof Coffee

1. Brew 2 tablespoon of freshly ground coffee. You can use French press to filter it
2. Add 1 or 2 tablespoon of grassfed butter or grassfed ghee or MCTs
3. Add 1 or 2 tablespoon of Organic Virgin Coconut oil
4. Add ½ teaspoon of freshly ground cinnamon or vanilla for flavor
5. Mix it all in a blender (We recommend the Nutri Bullet Blender) for less than a minute or until it gets a foamy texture and looks like a latte.

Teas: I like Rooibos tea that is known to increase AMPK. It is also caffeine free for those who want to avoid caffeine. Green tea and black tea will also increase AMPK levels and are good beverages.

Drinking 5 or more cups of coffee per day lowers risk of diabetes by 50%.

---

94. DIABETES AND ALCOHOL

Ethanol is made by fermenting sugar. Beer and sweet wines especially will raise blood sugar.

Alcohol can affect diabetes in several ways.

1. Hypoglycemia in diabetes from excess alcohol.
2. Stimulates appetite and causes you to overeat.
3. Alcohol (especially mixed drinks) will increase weight.
4. Alcohol can affect your judgment causing poor food choices.
5. Alcohol can interfere with insulin.
6. Alcohol may increase blood pressure.
7. Excess alcohol can damage both the pancreas and liver.
8. Alcohol can alter your microbiome negatively.
9. Alcohol from wheat may aggravate 'gluten sensitivity'.
10. Alcohol (especially beer) can cause acute gout.

Simple Rules

- Limit alcohol to 1 glass of wine for a female and 2 glasses for a male.
- Avoid desert wines (20gm/carbs/glass).
- Avoid beer (12gm carb) compared to wine (4-5gm/glass).
- Vodka, gin, rum, and whisky have little or no carbs (beware of mixers).
- Never add juices (28gm carbs) as a mixer.
- Don't add "diet sodas" as a mixer; they damage your microbiome.
- If you do drink a beer, occasionally choose a "light beer".

Remember, the body will burn alcohol before even sugar, so that you have now placed another barrier that prevents your body burning your fat stores. Only 20% of the alcohol you drink gets metabolized – 80% goes straight to the liver that cause DNL like fructose causing insulin resistance.

**One or two glasses of red wine (full of antioxidants)
is your best choice if you choose to drink alcohol.**

---

95. THE IMPORTANCE OF NUTRITION AND METABOLISM

An old Chinese proverb states that, "He that takes medication and neglects diet wastes the time of his physician."

The whole purpose of this short book is to help empower you to reverse (cure) your diabetes which as you have seen is a completely reversible disease with the information you have in your hands (not from the advice of the ADA).

- Avoid all processed food, especially sugar, grains and trans fats which cause most chronic disease.

- Eat a Keto (HFLC) Diet: meat, poultry, fish, eggs, vegetables, salads, friendly fruits and nuts.

- Avoid all wheat and grains: No breads, cakes, muffins, pancakes, or cereals.

- Try Intermittent Fasting (IF). I like the 16/8 IF which just means eat dinner early and breakfast late. Try to confine eating to the 8 hours window and limit carbs to less 50gm/day.

- Do not heat plant oils; cook only with butter, ghee, lard, or coconut oil (olive oil on salads is great).

- Avoid diet sodas and artificial sweeteners of all kinds.

- Avoid skim and low fat milk. Use full fat (LOW FAT = HIGH SUGAR).

- Limit alcohol to 1-2 drinks per day (No BEER, or mixed drinks).

- Avoid fruit juice and sodas (coffee and tea are fine).

Three of the most important measurements to assess your nutrition and metabolism are Waist-Stature ratio, Percent Body Fat, and HbA1c.

---

96. HIGH GLYCEMIC LOAD FOODS TO AVOID

FOOD GROUP	HIGH GLYCEMIC LOAD
Fruits	Tropical Fruits, Fruit Juices and Drinks
Dairy	Sweetened Yogurt, Whey Protein (20% people)
Grains	Bread, highly processed (including bagels, buns, corn, bread, English muffin, peas rolls, and white bread)
	Breakfast cereals, low fiber
	Couscous
	Crackers
	Pancakes
	Pasta
	Pizza
	Popcorn
	Pretzels
	Rice Cakes
	Stuffing
	Taco Shell
	Tortilla
	Waffle
	White Rice
Desserts, Sweets, & Treats	Brownies
	Cake
	Candy
	Chips
	Cookies
	Custards
	Doughnuts
	Pies
	Sorbet
	Sugary Drinks

Note: Grains and desserts (sugar) have the highest glycemic load and must be avoided to reduce diabesity. (Fat and Protein have little or no effect on GL.)

---

4 Week Diabetis Cure · Graham Simpson MD

97. FRUITS TO EAT AND FRUITS TO AVOID

Remember, fruit is nature's candy and they are high in fructose which is toxic and should be avoided or kept to a minimum if you have diabetes.

Best fruits are those that have less than 5gm fructose per serving.

FRUITS TO EAT

FRUIT	SERVING SIZE	GRAMS OF FRUCTOSE
Avocado	Unlimited	0
Limes	1 medium	0
Lemons	1 medium	0.6
Cranberries	1 cup	0.7
Passion Fruit	1 medium	0.9
Prune	1 medium	1.2
Apricot	1 medium	1.3
Guava	2 medium	2.2
Date (Deglet Noor style)	1 medium	2.6
Cantaloupe	1/8 of med. Melon	2.8
Raspberries	1 cup	3
Clementine	1 medium	3.4
Kiwi Fruit	1 medium	3.4
Blackberries	1 cup	3.5
Star Fruit	1 medium	3.6
Cherries, sweet	10	3.8
Strawberries	1 cup	3.8
Cherries, sour	1 cup	4
Pineapple	1 slice (3.5" x .75")	4
Grapefruit, pink or red	1/2 medium	4.3

FRUITS TO AVOID

FRUIT	SERVING SIZE	GRAMS OF FRUCTOSE
Boysenberries	1 cup	4.6
Tangerine/	1 medium	0
mandarin orange	1 medium	4.8
Nectarine	1 medium	5.4
Peach	1 medium	5.9
Orange (navel)	1 medium	6.1
Papaya	1/2 medium	6.3
Honeydew	1/8 of med. melon	6.7
Banana	1 medium	7.1
Blueberries	1 cup	7.4
Date (Medjool)	1 medium	7.7
Apple (composite)	1 medium	9.5
Persimmon	1 medium	10.6
Watermelon	1 1/6 med. Melon	11.3
Pear	1 medium	11.8
Raisins	1/4 cup	12.3
Grape, seedless (green or red)	1 cup	12.4
Mango	1/2 medium	16.2
Apricots, dried	1 cup	16.4
Figs, dried	1 cup	23

Adapted from Always Hungry, David Ludwig MD

If you have autoimmune disease like diabetes, only eat avocado, green mangos, green bananas and green papaya.

---

98. OIL AND VINEGAR BEST DRESSING FOR DIABESITY

Vinegar is derived from the Latin 'vinum acer' which means sour wine (acetic acid). Vinegar has been used as a cleaning agent, antibiotic, preservative and in our salad dressings.

Diluted vinegar is also a tonic for weight loss. Apple cider vinegar has both acetic acid and pectin from apples.

The Romans were one of the earliest cultures to use vinegar to treat diabetes. Vinegar seems to improve insulin resistance. Two teaspoons of vinegar taken with a high carb meal lowers blood sugar and insulin as much as 34%.

I encourage clients to use a 3:1 mixture of virgin olive oil to 1 tablespoon of balsamic vinegar as the perfect salad dressing. Even when potatoes are served cold, if vinegar is added it lowers the glycemic index.

Vinegar appears to exert a protective effect on the serum insulin response.

Health Benefits of Olive Oil

Lowers Risk of:

- Heart Disease
- Cancer
- Oxidative Stress (polyphenols)
- Inflammation
- Diabetes
- Blood Pressure
- Obesity
- Alzheimers
- Rheumatoid Arthritis
- Osteoporosis

Health Benefits of Vinegar

- Lowers blood sugar
- Improves blood circulation
- Packed with antioxidants
- Aids in weight loss
- Aids in digestion
- Cleaning agent
- Antibiotic properties

Type II diabetics who take 2 tablespoons of apple cider vinegar in water at bedtime reduce their fasting morning sugars.

How vinegar produces its health benefits is not clear. It might inhibit starches or reduce the speed of gastric emptying.

The use of oil and vinegar dressings on salads have been shown not only to help insulin resistance but also cause less cardiovascular disease.

Use generous amounts of olive oil and vinegar on salads.

---

99. THE ROLE OF BARIATRIC SURGERY IN DIABETES

There is now overwhelming evidence that diabetes and morbidly obese clients can be cured with Bariatric Surgery. In fact, many insurance companies will now cover this procedure as they recognize the potential cost savings.

Bariatric Surgery also proves that diabetes can be cured!

In an article in Lancet in 1925, it was reported that partial removal of the stomach for peptic ulcer disease often caused weight loss and resolution of diabetes.

Jejunocolic bypass and Jejunoileal bypass surgeries were performed with the later Rou-En-Y gastric procedure becoming the common form of Bariatric surgery today.

An even simpler procedure is the "sleeve gastrectomy" and "gastric lap band" that produce milder weight loss with fewer side effects. More recently a simple procedure using a balloon that can be inflated avoids surgery.

Many organizations recommend bariatric surgery as the first line therapy for type II diabetes with a body mass over 40.

With the sudden severe calorie restriction, the body depletes its liver glycogen stores within 24hrs and begins burning fat. The first fat burnt is the visceral and ectopic fat that reverses diabetes long before there is any obvious weight loss.

As insulin secretion returns to normal (removing the ectopic fat from the pancreas resolves the Beta cell dysfunction), blood glucose drops. Removing the fat from the liver reverses the insulin resistance.

A simple Keto-Diet and I.F. will do the same safely.

Surgery is expensive and may cause many complications.

**All Bariatric Surgeries are effective as they
create a sudden severe calorie reduction.**

---

100. HOW TO LIVE TO A HUNDRED

Metabolic and Psychological Stress is what shortens our telomeres and our lives. With aging, the DNA of our cells become progressively damaged causing cells to become irreversibly aged and dysfunctional.

Telomeres throughout the body shorten with aging (telomerase, the enzyme responsible for restoring DNA, is lost during cell division) and contributes to cardio-metabolic disease and faster aging. We want to "Eat right, Stay Fit, Live Long, Die Quick."

Metabolic Stress

Diabetes and insulin resistance is the prototypical disease for aging. We have several remedies.

- A **HFLC Keto diet** can increase our lifespan by 7-10 years (UC Davis).
- **Exercise** can increase our telomeres adding 7 years to our life (PLOS).
- **Fasting** can increase the human life by 8 years (UCSD).
- Any factor **increasing AMPK** e.g. Metformin will increase lifespan (#72).
- Any factor **decreasing MTOR** e.g. Rapamycin will increase lifespan (#73).
- **Minimize toxins** e.g. Life expectancy for smokers 10 years shorter than non-smokers (WHO).
- **Hormone Optimization** e.g. Lower IgF1 by reducing sugar and animal protein extend life (USCD).
- **Adequate Supplements** e.g. Vit D3 and Vit K2 and many others extend life (Life Extension).
- **Gut Health** e.g. Certain nutrients and probiotics extend longevity 60% in fruit flies (McGill Univ) and probably in humans.
- **Senolytics** e.g. Fisetin (flavonoid) destroys senescent cells reducing inflammation and increasing longevity.

Psychological Stress

Studies have shown that people with the highest levels of stress have telomere shortening an average of 10 years compared to lower stressed individuals. Increase in all cardio-metabolic disease is evident. Psychological stress promotes regulatory changes important in ageing – increased stress hormones, inflammation, oxidative stress, and hyperinsulinemia. In addition, there is lower telomerase activity and shorter telomere length known determinants of cell senescence and longevity. (UCLA Article)

Be sure to reduce both metabolic and psychological stress.

Afterword

The Program: Four Week Diabetes Cure (eternityonline.com)

Definition: Reverse Diabetes

Reversing Diabetes is a term that usually refers to a significant long term improvement in "insulin sensitivity" in people with type II diabetes.

People with type II diabetes, who are able to get their HbA1c below 6.4 without medication, are said to have reversed or resolved their diabetes (remission).

Definition: Cure Diabetes

A cure is a methodology that ends a medical condition, such as diabetes or prediabetes (HbA1c <5.7), that helps end a person's suffering (that state of being healed) by removing all its root-causes.

Half of the world now has diabetes or prediabetes. We believe that the majority of people with Heart disease, Cancer, and Alzheimer's have 'insulin resistance' that causes not only Diabetes, but in fact most of the chronic disease that afflicts us today.

We will not, as I have shown, cure type II diabetes by following the American Diabetes Association (ADA) nutritional guidelines, taking insulin or oral hypoglycemic drugs.

Let us prove to you what we promise. The first step is to contact us and have a painless Blood Sugar Sensor placed on your arm that will measure your sugar levels every 15min, 96 times a day for 2 weeks. We will then demonstrate to you: it is not only "what you eat" but also "when you eat" that counts. We promise delicious, natural, real food, and that you will never be hungry as you begin to reverse and cure your diabetes and obesity. Awareness changes behavior.

We provide a 'whole person' approach that is personalized, aimed at those key factors that are causing your "insulin resistance." As many people with type II diabetes are also overweight (Diabesity), you will also lose weight with your program without feeling tired and hungry. You should remain Keto or Paleo for the rest of your life which is not difficult to do. The program is safe and based on the latest nutritional science shown to produce proven positive outcomes in the large majority of individuals.

We use an Online Integral Health Model with a simple 3 step approach:

Step 1 Measure: We do a comprehensive history, examination, and select diagnostics.

Step 2 Mentor: We use the INTEGRAL acronym shown below to find the root-cause of your problem and then reverse it.

ROOT CAUSE
Inflammation
Nutrition
Toxins
Exercise/Sleep
Gut Microbiome
Restoration of Hormones
Adequate Supplements
Lifetime Mindfulness (Stress Reduction)

Step 3 Monitor: We encourage you to select one of our online certified health coaches and doctors who will monitor you with the Eternity APP, especially over the first few weeks when we will be reducing your medications.

Most often, after the first month and once you are 'in the flow' with your new WFKD, you will need less monitoring by our coaches and physicians.

Our medical personnel are always ready to assist you with any issues, questions, or problems you may have.

All products you need can be shipped to you anywhere in the world.

As Jason Fung, MD points out, there have been many large successful trials that have shown that lifestyle interventions (not drugs) can reverse and also prevent diabetes. For example:

1. China Da Qing Diabetes Prevention Outcome Study
The main intervention – increase vegetables and decrease sugar and alcohol.
- reduced incidence of diabetes by 43% (sustained over 20 years)
- cardiovascular death rate fell from 20% to 1%

2. Diabetes Prevention Program in the USA
- reduced incidence diabetes by 58% (sustained for 10 years)

3. Indian Diabetes Prevention Program
- reduced incidence diabetes by 30%

4. Finnish Diabetes Prevention Study
- reduced incidence diabetes by 58%

5. Japanese Study on Diabetes Prevention
- reduced progression of diabetes by 67%

6. Virta (2018) Study in USA
- reversed diabetes in more than 60% diabetics – most within just two months (done remotely).

7. DHA (Dubai) Study
- We will publish DATA end 2019

8. Dabur (India) Study
- We will publish DATA end 2019

The important common factor is that all of these studies used simple lifestyle interventions – not drugs to reverse and prevent diabetes.

It is important to recognize that you hold in your hands 100 simple facts that can help cure your diabesity for good! Please contact eternityonline for your Diabesity APP today and begin to reverse your disease.

May You Live Healthy and Happy

Testimonials

Francisco M. Torres, MD
Florida,USA

Thank you Dr. Graham Simpson, my age management medicine mentor.

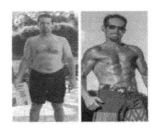

I would like to thank publicly Dr. Simpson. I reconnected with him while in Dubai seven years after my initial training with him. I will be forever grateful for all he taught me in the field of age management medicine. Both the knowledge and practical application of this knowledge have been a great help and support to me through this amazing journey. I believe my success is due in part to his sincere support and mentorship. I want to therefore express my deepest gratitude to Dr. Simpson for giving me this priceless opportunity. His support will forever remain a major contributor behind my success and achievements in this field of medicine.

Dion Friedland
IBFA Mr. Europe and Mr. Universe(Age Category 70+) South Africa

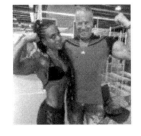

I met Dr. Graham Simpson 14 years ago while on vacation in the Caribbean and was introduced to Anti-Aging medicine by him. As a result I have been able to dramatically improve my health and appearance since then by following a Keto/Paleo styled diet, judicious hormone replacement, regular exercise in gyms and select nutraceuticals. My body fat percent has dropped from the mid 20's to 5% – 7%. I recently won the IBFF World Body Building Championships 70 and over (I'm 75 yrs old); the IBFA Mr. Universe and Mr. Europe 70 and over and intend continuing this lifestyle until they put me in a box. I have more energy and feel and look better than when in my forties. I have no reservation in recommending Dr Simpson's Proactive lifestyle program to transform your health too and guarantee that if you follow his advice you will have more energy and will look and feel many years younger.

Jacob Rosenstein MD
Arlington Texas, USA

My partner and I met Dr. Simpson at Cenegenics Institute in Las Vegas where we received training from him. After following his advice on a HFLC diet for 8 months, I was able to drop my body fat over 10%, reversed my pre-diabetes and felt renewed. Although I am a neurosurgeon, I added the S.W. Age Intervention Program and have helped hundreds of patients regain their metabolic health and vitality.

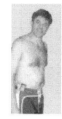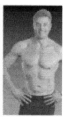

Nancy Flocchini
Director of Human Resources, AT&T Nevada, USA

The day I walked into the Center and started my age management program, my blood sugars were running over 600. I was taking five shots of insulin per day, my vision was disappearing, and I had no energy. After approximately eight months on a Keto/Paleo diet, my blood sugars are now consistently around 85 and I no longer take any insulin shots. My cholesterol has gone from 353 to 166 and my triglycerides have gone from 442 to 110. Plus, I've lost an incredible 80 pounds and I have my energy back. My endocrinologist is flabbergasted. Thank you, Dr. Simpson, for changing my life.

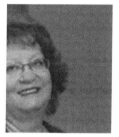

Wasim Akram
Karachi, Pakistan
Former Captain of the Pakistan Cricket Team

I met Dr. Simpson at Eternity more than five years ago. As most people know I have had diabetes for many years. Since following a High Fat Low Carb (HFLC) diet and select nutraceuticals and a more balanced lifestyle I'm pleased to say that the Eternity Metabolic Center's whole person approach has made a significant improvement to my diabetes, energy and overall sense of wellbeing. I believe a WFKD can also benefit those with Type I Diabetes.

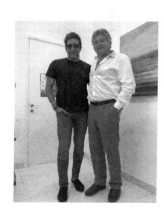

Deepak Pal
Delhi, India

My name is Deepak Pal. I have been eating a Keto and Paleo diet for the last 10 months since I met Dr. Simpson. I'm a 29 year old. I was 84kg before I got into this diet. But in 3 months I was getting results. What's more I am a complete vegetarian and I want to let all of you know that a Paleo-Vegetarian diet is easy. My energy levels are going up. My weight is dropping slowly, but surely (it is now 67kg). My skin looks 10 years younger. I feel better than I have in years. This is no longer a 'diet'. It's a new way of life. I won't go back. I will look forward to my feeling good/healthy future with a Keto and Paleo Lifestyle.

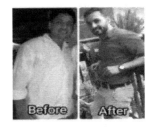

Resources

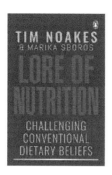 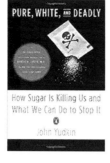 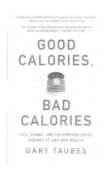 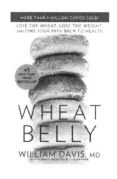

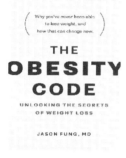 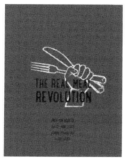 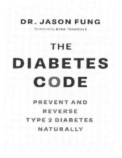 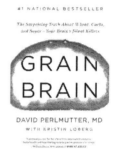

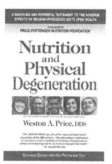 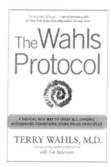 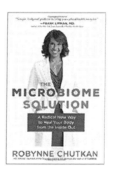 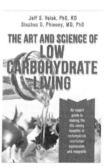

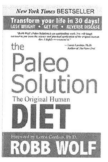 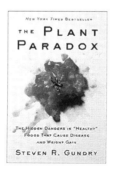 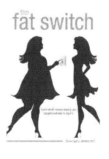 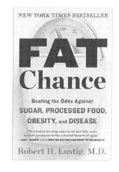

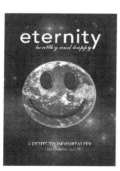 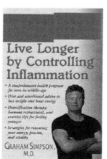 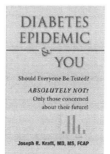 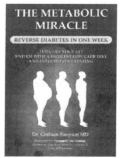

Made in the USA
Lexington, KY
06 July 2019